OBSTETRICS AND GYNECOLOGY ADVANCES

INFERTILITY

GENETIC FACTORS, TREATMENT RISKS AND BENEFITS, SOCIAL AND PSYCHOLOGICAL CONSEQUENCES

OBSTETRICS AND GYNECOLOGY ADVANCES

Additional books in this series can be found on Nova's website under the Series tab.

Additional E-books in this series can be found on Nova's website under the E-book tab.

HUMAN REPRODUCTIVE SYSTEM - ANATOMY, ROLES AND DISORDERS

Additional books in this series can be found on Nova's website under the Series tab.

Additional E-books in this series can be found on Nova's website under the E-book tab.

OBSTETRICS AND GYNECOLOGY ADVANCES

INFERTILITY

GENETIC FACTORS, TREATMENT RISKS AND BENEFITS, SOCIAL AND PSYCHOLOGICAL CONSEQUENCES

RENATO NASCIMENTO
AND
HENRIQUE VILAS BOAS
EDITORS

New York

For permission to use material from this book please contact us:
Telephone 631-231-7269; Fax 631-231-8175
Web Site: http://www.novapublishers.com

Library of Congress Cataloging-in-Publication Data

ISBN: 978-1-62257-909-9

Library of Congress Control Number: 2012947890

Published by Nova Science Publishers, Inc. † New York

Contents

Preface

Infertility affects about 15% of couples in western societies. In addition to isolation, infertility challenges women's sense of identity, expectations of their life trajectory and their perceived value in society. This book presents current research on the genetic factors, treatment risk and benefits, and social and psychological consequences of infertility. Topics include the traditional Chinese medicine approach to fertility management; adverse outcomes of assisted reproduction techniques; the impact of follicular fluid components and embryo-endometrial cross-talk on the oocyte quality or embryo viability; iatrogenic damage incurred during fertility treatment upon gamete competence and embryonic viability; genetic factors of male infertility; animal models for studying female infertility; and treatment of endometriosis associated with infertility.

Chapter 1 - Infertility affects about 15% of couples in western societies. Despite infertility occurring relatively often in the population, it is experienced as a lonely road for individual couples. In addition to isolation, infertility challenges women's sense of identity, expectations of their life trajectory and their perceived value in society. This can lead to feelings of failure, guilt and shame. Women's sense of powerlessness can be exacerbated by the Western medical approach, through fragmented care, technical interventions and invasive procedures, and a lack of individualised continuous support.

Infertility may be experienced for several years and the draining becomes more considerable with time. While some help is offered through the Western medical health system via in-vitro- fertilisation (IVF), IVF procedures are expensive, often painful, physically and emotionally, with only 18% resulting in live births. Traditional Chinese Medicine (TCM) offers holistic non-invasive treatment options for infertility with a higher success rate of up to 60% resulting in life births. However, awareness about TCM and the menstrual cycle as a diagnostic tool is low amongst women, couples, as well as medical doctors.

Part 1 of this chapter summarises current evidence of the effect of Traditional Chinese Herbal Medicine in the management of female infertility and on pregnancy rates compared with Western Medical drug treatment based on the authors' systematic review and meta-analysis.

Part 2 of this chapter provides an overview of menstrual cycle characteristics and their relation to fertility status, providing a non-invasive diagnostic tool routinely used in the Traditional Chinese Medicine approach to general health and fertility.

Part 3 and 4 tell the stories of ten women with infertility in their own voices who had sought Traditional Chinese Medicine therapy captured by interview. Some women had problems conceiving, some had suffered miscarriages or stillbirths, most had been told that their infertility was 'unexplained'. Women shared their journey of trying to achieve a viable pregnancy, some for as long as 10 years, what they did, how they felt, how they coped. They reveal where they found support, empowerment and importantly, hope.

All women agreed that awareness and recognition of holistic therapies such as Traditional Chinese Medicine (TCM) in relation to fertility is low, and wished to raise awareness and help other women by telling their story. Each of the women's stories is unique including the reasons for infertility, how they navigated the health system, what support they had and how they coped. Their stories display the diversity of infertility and treatment approaches, and shed light on relevant lifestyle and environmental factors, as well as menstrual health, often dismissed in a conventional medical diagnosis.

Chapter 2 - From the first birth of a child conceived by in vitro fertilization (IVF), much has been developed in assisted reproduction techniques (ART). However, the evolution of knowledge and therapeutic options, and progressively better results, were not followed by a proper control of risks and complications, which are still considerably frequent. The aim of this chapter is to deeply discuss undesirable outcomes such as ovarian hyperstimulation syndrome, ectopic and multiple pregnancies, and the higher rates of miscarriage among patients submitted to ART. In addition, birth defects, epigenetic inheritance and perinatal outcomes will be discussed, with the aim to offer clinicians an updated reference for daily practice.

Chapter 3 - To overcome the still insufficient implantation rate following *in vitro* fertilization (IVF) in humans, more than two embryos are commonly replaced which potentially leads to a high number of multiple pregnancies with associated risks such as low birth weight. The solution for avoiding multiple pregnancies could be optimalization of embryo selection and single embryo transfer. The traditional systems for assessing gamete and embryo viability have limited ability to accurately select those with the best developmental potential. Morphological evaluation remains the primary method of oocyte and embryo assessment during IVF cycles. However, its modest predictive power and inherent inter- and intra-observer variability limits its clinical value. Prolonged embryo culture to blastocyst stage was introduced as a possible strategy for selecting the best embryos but the extended period of *in vitro* culture may have its side effects.

Successful embryo implantation requires accurate temporal regulation of maternal immune functions to accommodate a semi-allogeneic embryo. To prepare the immunological tolerance at the beginning of implantation, the precise temporal regulations between the immune and endocrine components are required. The authors' review will focus on molecules of embryo-endometrial cross-talk that are engaged in regulation of the embryo implantation, and on selected follicular fluid components that might play a role in developmental/embryogenic potential of the oocyte. The review will also discuss advances in the understanding of the regulation of fertility that has been made during last 15 years with the production of over 400 mutant mouse models with a reproductive phenotype. Indeed, the past few years have witnessed a virtual explosion in the identification of gene mutations or polymorphisms that cause or are linked to human infertility and that are inherited in a polygenic/multifactorial fashion. The aim of this review is to point out two recent trends in reproductive medicine - the search for potentially useful biomarkers for improvement of pregnancy rates after the assisted reproduction techniques (ART); and the importance of homeostasis that makes spontaneous conception possible. Especially in diagnoses like the endometriosis, the causes of infertility remains not fully understood and the best option for these patients is a return to the balance that enables the spontaneous conception.

Chapter 4 - Infertility affects an estimated 9% of couples worldwide. While advances in assisted reproductive technology (ART) have revolutionised the treatment of infertility, success rates are highly variable. Pregnancy and delivery rates for common techniques such as *in vitro* fertilisation (IVF) and intracytoplasmic sperm injection (ICSI) rarely exceed 30% and 23% respectively. An increasing body of evidence strongly suggests that routine ART techniques may inadvertently induce detrimental effects upon gametes and embryos, compromising either gamete fertility or embryonic viability. Consequently, it is critical that ART protocols are constantly refined or replaced in line with scientific advances, such that clinics can provide patients with an optimised chance of successful conception. Here, the authors discuss a number of ways in which ART protocols are known to induce detrimental effect upon critical biomarkers of gamete and embryo health, and identify future areas for investigative research. As the number of couples seeking fertility treatment worldwide increases, the efficacy of ART is more important than ever. By informing the research community of the potential ways in which ART may compromise gamete and embryo viability, it is the intention of this commentary to inspire concerted research effort such that ART protocols can be refined or replaced as necessary.

Chapter 5 – The authors' understanding of genomic medicine has increased with developments in molecular biology, stem cell technology, and research on the DNA content of the human genome. Advances in these areas have had considerable impact on the field of genetic male infertility. Many causes of genetic male infertility have been extensively studied, including Klinefelter syndrome (47, XXY), chromosomal aneuploidies, chromosomal translocation, Y-chromosome microdeletions, X-chromosome abnormalities, single-gene defects, and abnormalities in DNA mismatch repair. However, many genetic abnormalities that result in male infertility are still unknown. Indeed, it is likely that most cases of male infertility have a definable underlying genetic cause. A better understanding of the genetic basis of infertility will lead to improvements in its diagnosis and treatment.

Chapter 6 - Female reproductive dysfunction accounts for about 40% of all human infertility cases. Although the molecular aspects of these disorders are still to be determined, the use of animal models over the last decade has shown itself to be a powerful tool in the understanding of female infertility. The development of knock-out and transgenic technology in the last few years has generated more than 300 different mice models that display reproductive defects. In the context of the study of female reproductive biology, the analysis of knock-out and transgenic mice has strongly contributed to clarify the underlying processes leading to follicular development, oocyte maturation, fertilization events or embryo implantation. This chapter provides a comprehensive compilation of the most relevant studies published in this area, from the early pioneering studies to the most recent developments, highlighting how the use of animal models can help us to understand the female reproductive system and the etiology of some female infertile disorders.

Chapter 7 - Despite the significant heterogeneity in the clinical manifestations of endometriosis, a high prevalence of the disease is observed in infertile women, and in women with chronic pelvic pain. The socioeconomic impact of this enigmatic condition is high, and the data regarding the efficacy of the different therapeutic approaches is quite conflicting.

Thus, the objective of this article is to describe the scientific evidence available regarding therapeutic modalities, and to provide recommendations for the treatment of infertility and chronic pelvic pain related to endometriosis. In patients with mild endometriosis, the suppression of ovarian function does not improve fertility, but the ablation of the lesions associated with adhesiolysis does seem to be more effective in improving fertility than the exclusive use of diagnostic laparoscopy.

There is insufficient evidence to determine whether surgical excision improves pregnancy rates in cases of moderate or severe endometriosis. In vitro fertilization (IVF) seems to be an adequate approach, especially in cases that involve other infertility factors and/or the failure of other treatments.

The use of GnRH for 3 to 6 months before IVF is recommended. With regard to pain relief, the suppression of ovarian function for 3 to 6 months in patients, whose endometriosis is laparoscopically confirmed, has been shown to reduce the pain associated with endometriosis. All of the medications studied seem to have similar efficacy, varying only in terms of adverse effects and cost. The ablation of endometriotic lesions reduces the pain associated with endometriosis, but is less effective in less severe cases of the disease.

The excision of endometriomas > 4 cm in diameter seems to improve the rate of natural fecundity, as well as the fertility rate obtained with assisted reproduction procedures. These procedures also reduce the levels of pain and the risk of recurrence. Finally, it is important to emphasize that there are countless controversies regarding the treatment of this disease, and that the recommendations described above should be revised as randomized controlled clinical trials with adequate patient enrollment generate evidence that is more reliable.

In: Infertility
Editors: R. Nascimento and H. V. Boas

ISBN: 978-1-62257-909-9

Chapter 1

Infertility: The Traditional Chinese Medicine Approach to Fertility Management, Menstrual Health, Fertility Awareness and Emotional Well-being

Karin Ried*
National Institute of Integrative Medicine, Victoria, Australia;
Discipline of General Practice, The University of Adelaide, South Australia

Abstract

Infertility affects about 15% of couples in western societies. Despite infertility occurring relatively often in the population, it is experienced as a lonely road for individual couples. In addition to isolation, infertility challenges women's sense of identity, expectations of their life trajectory and their perceived value in society. This can lead to feelings of failure, guilt and shame. Women's sense of powerlessness can be exacerbated by the Western medical approach, through fragmented care, technical interventions and invasive procedures, and a lack of individualised continuous support.

Infertility may be experienced for several years and the draining becomes more considerable with time. While some help is offered through the Western medical health system via in-vitro- fertilisation (IVF), IVF procedures are expensive, often painful, physically and emotionally, with only 18% resulting in live births. Traditional Chinese Medicine (TCM) offers holistic non-invasive treatment options for infertility with a higher success rate of up to 60% resulting in life births. However, awareness about TCM and the menstrual cycle as a diagnostic tool is low amongst women, couples, as well as medical doctors.

Part 1 of this chapter summarises current evidence of the effect of Traditional Chinese Herbal Medicine in the management of female infertility and on pregnancy rates

* Email: karinried@niim.com.au; karin.ried@adelaide.edu.au.

compared with Western Medical drug treatment based on our systematic review and meta-analysis.

Part 2 of this chapter provides an overview of menstrual cycle characteristics and their relation to fertility status, providing a non-invasive diagnostic tool routinely used in the Traditional Chinese Medicine approach to general health and fertility.

Part 3 and 4 tell the stories of ten women with infertility in their own voices who had sought Traditional Chinese Medicine therapy captured by interview. Some women had problems conceiving, some had suffered miscarriages or stillbirths, most had been told that their infertility was 'unexplained'. Women shared their journey of trying to achieve a viable pregnancy, some for as long as 10 years, what they did, how they felt, how they coped. They reveal where they found support, empowerment and importantly, hope.

All women agreed that awareness and recognition of holistic therapies such as Traditional Chinese Medicine (TCM) in relation to fertility is low, and wished to raise awareness and help other women by telling their story. Each of the women's stories is unique including the reasons for infertility, how they navigated the health system, what support they had and how they coped. Their stories display the diversity of infertility and treatment approaches, and shed light on relevant lifestyle and environmental factors, as well as menstrual health, often dismissed in a conventional medical diagnosis.

Introduction

Infertility affects 15% or 3 million of couples in Australia and is defined as the inability to conceive or achieve a viable pregnancy after one year of regular unprotected intercourse. While 80% of infertility might be related to conditions such as endometriosis or Polycystic Ovary Syndrome (PCOS), 20% are 'unexplained' in the Western Medicine model [1, 2]. However, diagnosis of a specific disease/condition and subsequent treatment with surgery, drugs, In-Vitro-Fertilisation (IVF) or other Assisted Reproductive Technologies (ART) does not always result in a viable pregnancy and live birth. In 2009, for example, more than 70,500 ART cycles were recorded in Australia and New Zealand, and only 17.2% resulted in live births [3].

Moreover, ART treatment is costly for both government and individuals; in 2009, the Australian Government spent approximately A$250 million for ART services [4], and individual couples' out-of-pocket expenses were about A$3,000 for one IVF cycle costing A$7,000-8,000 [5].

Infertility causes emotional distress and grief for the affected couple [6, 7]. However, there is a lack of recognition by organisations and the community for couples suffering infertility or recurrent miscarriages, and support services are inferior to those offered for a visible loss of pregnancy such as stillbirth [8-11].

Alternative holistic therapies, such as Traditional Chinese Medicine, offer less invasive and less costly physical and emotional treatment compared with standard Western Medical treatment. However, awareness of TCM therapy for infertility is generally low and often not suggested by Western medical practitioners [11, 12]. The first port of call for most couples experiencing infertility in Australia are general practitioners, who routinely refer to infertility clinics for initial investigations and potential IVF treatment [13].

Traditional Chinese Medicine searches for the individual's underlying imbalances causing the infertility using diagnostic tools such as pulse, tongue, complexion, general physical and emotional wellbeing, and menstrual history. TCM pattern diagnosis determines the specific individual treatment including Chinese Herbal Medicine (CHM) and acupuncture. TCM pattern diagnosis refers to whole body systems such as meridians and involves the Kidney, Liver (Blood), Spleen, Heart, and Lung systems, excess or deficiency patterns, heat or cold patterns. The treatment principle in TCM is to balance any diagnosed imbalance [14-18].

A thorough assessment of menstrual history is embedded in standard TCM pattern diagnosis in female infertility, providing a visible window into the woman's (in-) fertility status. The combination of the basal body temperature (BBT) curve, menstrual flow, colour of the menstrual blood and clot formation, mucus changes, and any associated pain or distension are directly related to TCM pattern diagnosis and therefore therapy [16, 19].

Part 1: Meta-analyses of the Effect of Traditional Chinese Herbal Medicine versus Western Medicine in the Management of Infertility

We undertook a meta-analysis of randomised controlled trials (RCT) as well as a meta-analysis of cohort studies that investigated the treatment of infertility with Traditional Chinese Herbal therapy [20]. Participants were women of reproductive age with primary or secondary infertility. Infertility may have been associated with endometriosis, PCOS, amenorrhea, advanced maternal age, or unexplained infertility. Our review excluded studies of male infertility.

Chinese Herbal Medicine (CHM) treatment was defined as treatment with Chinese Herbs according to TCM pattern diagnosis. We included studies which used CHM alone or in combination with acupuncture or Western Medicine (WM) in the form of drugs or surgery. The control group in RCTs received WM pharmacological treatment only. We excluded studies using acupuncture alone or TCM therapy in combination with assisted reproductive technologies (ART).

The primary outcome was clinical pregnancy. We also assessed infertility status (number of years unsuccessful in achieving viable pregnancy), maternal age, CHM treatment duration, WM condition, and TCM pattern diagnosis, and - if available - live birth rate.

We used the Cochrane Review methodology and program to select studies of sufficient quality for analysis [21].

In addition, we related common TCM pattern diagnosis in infertility to the quality of the menstrual cycle (colour, consistency and flow of blood, frequency, BBT, and associated symptoms including pain), and tongue and pulse appearance.

Characteristics of studies included in the meta-analyses are described in detail in Ried & Stuart (2011) [20]. In summary, women were between 18 and 45 years old, with a mean of 30 years. Infertility was experienced on average 4.5 years (range 1-20 years). Treatment duration with CHM was on average 4 months.

Study	TCM n	TCM N	Control n	Control N	Weight	Odds Ratio Random, 95% CI
Hua 03	50	76	8	31	11.7%	5.53 [2.17, 14.06]
Wu 06	32	48	29	52	13.8%	1.59 [0.70, 3.57]
Lin 05	34	48	12	42	12.0%	6.07 [2.43, 15.15]
Xia 04	24	46	9	40	11.6%	3.76 [1.47, 9.63]
Chen 95	19	60	6	25	9.8%	1.47 [0.50, 4.27]
Shao 04	21	32	11	30	10.1%	3.30 [1.16, 9.34]
Ren 02	17	28	11	30	9.9%	2.67 [0.92, 7.72]
Zhang 06	182	298	26	119	21.2%	5.61 [3.43, 9.19]
Total (95% CI)		**636**		**369**	**100.0%**	**3.50 [2.34, 5.24]**
Total events	379		112			

Heterogeneity: Tau² = 0.14; Chi² = 12.03, df = 7 (P = 0.10); I² = 42%

Test for overall effect: Z = 6.09 (P < 0.00001)

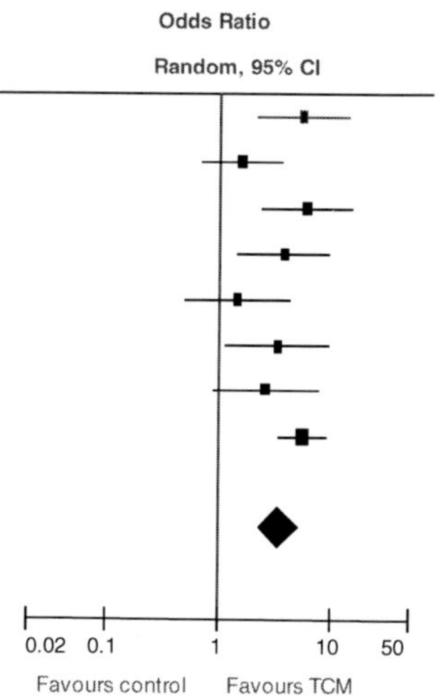

A) Meta-analysis of RCTs.

Study	n/N	ES (95% CI)	Weight (%)
Luolan 86	136/343	0.40 (0.34, 0.45)	55.68
Zhang 01	55/94	0.59 (0.48, 0.69)	15.26
Fang 91	18/32	0.56 (0.38, 0.74)	5.19
Wing 06	28/50	0.56 (0.41, 0.70)	8.12
Tan 01	30/41	0.73 (0.57, 0.86)	6.66
Tian 98	21/29	0.72 (0.53, 0.87)	4.71
Usuki 89	12/27	0.44 (0.25, 0.65)	4.38
Total	300/616	0.49 (0.45, 0.53)	100.00

Overall effect: I²= 82.8%, p < 0.0001

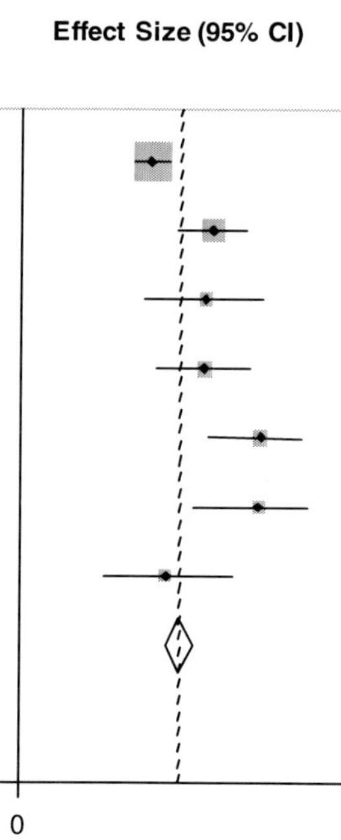

B) Adjusted meta-analysis of cohort studies.

Figure 1. (A) Meta-analysis of RCTs investigating pregnancy rates of infertile women treated with Chinese Herbal Medicine (CHM) compared with WM fertility medications, (B) Adjusted meta-analysis of cohort studies investigating pregnancy rates of infertile women treated with CHM.
TCM, Traditional Chinese Medicine; CI, confidence interval; n, number of pregnancies; N, number of women; ES, effect size.
Reprinted from Complementary Therapies in Medicine 19 (6), Ried K & Stuart K, 319-331, copyright (2011) with permission from Elsevier [20].

Meta-analysis of RCTs

The likelihood of achieving a pregnancy with CHM therapy over a 4-month period were 3.5 times higher (95%CI: 2.34, 5.24, p<0.0001) than with WM drug therapy in women with infertility (n=1005 in 8 RCTs). Mean pregnancy rates in the CHM group were 60% compared with 32% in the WM group (Figure 1a).

Meta-analysis of Cohort Studies

Most women participating in the cohort studies had primary infertility and had been diagnosed with a range of WM conditions including PCOS, endometriosis, oligomenorrhea, amenorrhea, dysmenorrhea, luteal phase defect, fallopian tube blockage, pelvic inflammation, hyperprolactinaemia, or unexplained infertility. The pooled pregnancy rate of seven high quality cohort studies included in the adjusted meta-analysis involving 616 women treated with CHM therapy was 48.7% (95%CI: 44.7, 52.7; Figure 1b).

The adjusted likelihood of achieving a pregnancy with CHM therapy ranging between 1 to 12 months were 2.3 higher (95%CI: 1.6, 3.4,p<0.0001) compared with the pregnancy rate of 30.4% in a cohort of women (n=7439) undergoing IVF in Australia in one year (2008/2009) [22].

Part 2: TCM Pattern Diagnosis and the Menstrual Cycle

In addition to pulse and tongue diagnosis, TCM uses the characteristics of the menstrual cycle as an essential diagnostic tool to ascertain underlying imbalances causing infertility.

The fundamental principle of TCM therapy is to restore balance within the body, which affects hormonal regulation of the menstrual cycle, and provides a physiological environment to facilitate conception, implantation, and maintenance of a viable pregnancy. The quality of the environment in the body is considered as important as the quality of eggs, sperm and embryo. TCM practitioners often refer to the environment, including the endometrium, as the 'soil' and eggs/embryo as the 'seed' (Chinese proverb: "Cultivate the soil before planting the seed") [14-18, 23]. Any irregularities in the menstrual cycle and general wellbeing, often seen in conditions associated with infertility, including advanced maternal age and unexplained infertility, are fundamental factors which can be optimised before conception is attempted [16, 17, 24].

We have summarised common TCM pattern diagnosis in infertility in relation to the quality of the menstrual cycle and associated symptoms, providing a practical guide to a woman's fertility status for health professionals but also women and couples experiencing infertility (Table 1, Figure 2).

The quality of the menstrual cycle is assessed by the appearance (colour, clots) and flow of the menstrual blood, the basal body temperature (BBT) curve, the length and frequency of the menstrual cycle, and the quality of the mucus during the cycle.

Table 1. Common TCM pattern in infertility and manifestations

TCM pattern	BBT	Quality of menses					Tongue	Pulse	Other symptoms	WM condition
		Colour	Clots	Flow	Frequency	Pain				
Kidney Jing Deficiency	Long follicular phase, low temp luteal phase; Unstable; monophasic, little fertile mucus	Pink, watery	No	Scanty	Delayed	Lower back	Pale	Weak thready	Low energy/ poor stamina, frequent urination, dark under eyes	Resistant ovary disease, ovarian failure, advanced ovarian age, amenorrhea
Kidney Yin deficiency	Short follicular phase, with higher temp (> 36.5°)	Bright red	No	Scanty	Irregular, shortened	Lower back, knees	Red with little coat, cracked	Thin, floating, rapid	Insomnia, dry throat /skin/ hair	PMS, amenorrhea, mild PCOS, premature menopause
Kidney Yang deficiency	Long follicular phase, low temp (≤ 36.2°); short luteal phase with low temp	Pale, light pink	Some times	Scanty	Irregular, delayed	Lower back, knees, legs	Pale, swollen	Deep, slow, weak	Pale complexion, fatigue, loose stools, feeling cold, low energy, low libido	Amenorrhea, insufficient progesterone
Spleen Qi deficiency	Slow-rise luteal phase (≥ 3 days, not usual 1-2 days); short luteal phase	Pink, watery	No	Scanty	Short	Mid-cycle pain	Swollen with white fur	Weak, slippery	Pale face, poor appetite, listlessness, loose stools	Amenorrhea, fibroids
Blood deficiency	Long follicular phase	Bright red	No	Scanty	Delayed	Mild lower abdominal, pressure relieves pain	Pale with little fur	Weak, deep, choppy	Dizziness, sallow complexion, fatigue, muscle spasm, brittle nails	Dysmenorrhea, amenorrhea, PCOS
Liver Qi Stagnation	Slow-rise unstable luteal phase	Dark red/ purple	Yes	Scanty	Irregular	Abdominal cramps	Dark red with purple spots	Deep wiry/ stringlike or choppy	Mood swings, irritability, headaches, breast distension	PMS, dysmenorrhea, irregular menstruation, amenorrhea
Heat, Kidney Yin deficiency	Follicular phase too short and temp too high	Dark red/ purple	Often	Heavy	Irregular, mid-cycle bleeding	Thick itchy leukorrhea	Red, peeled (sides, tip) with yellow coating	Thin, rapid, wiry	Red cheeks, hot palms/soles, hot flushes, insomnia,	May be associated with hyperactive thyroid, essential hypertension,

		Colour	Clots	Flow	Frequency	Pain				
									agitation, weight loss, constipation, thirst, nosebleed	menopausal symptoms
Liver or Heart Fire	Unstable follicular + luteal phase, sawtooth or saddle pattern	Dark red	Some times	Thick, excessive	Shortened, intermittent bleeding	Abdominal	Red tip	Rapid	Irritability, thirst, restless sleep, headache, red complexion	Metorrhagia/mid-cycle bleeding, PMS
Damp-heat	Monophasic, little fertile mucus	Dark red	No	Scanty, sticky thick, often maldorous	Irregular	Lower abdomen, loins, bloating	Red with thick, greasy yellow fur	Slippery, full, rapid	Dysbiosis in digestive system, no appetite, nausea	Infection, inflammation, endometritis, PID
Phlegm-damp Cold-damp	Long follicular phase, Monophasic temp chart	Dark	Yes	Scanty	Delayed	Abdominal distension, pain	Pale with white fur	Deep, fine, slow	Cold limbs, poor appetite, overweight, dull-pale complexion, congested throat, heaviness	Fallopian tube blockage, PCOS, ovarian cysts, amenorrhea, dysmenorrhea
Blood stasis & Dampness	Slow fall of temp at start of cycle	Dark purple	Yes	Heavy	Irregular	Lower abdominal	Purple swollen sticky coating	Wiry, slippery	Low energy, feeling cold, emotional stress, anxiety	Endometriosis, ovarian cysts, fibroids
Cold uterus	Low temp	Dark brown spotting	Some times	Scanty	Irregular	Painful periods	Pale, or purplish	Deep, weak, slow, wiry	Cold limbs, loose stools, frequent urination	Recurrent miscarriage

References: 15-19.

Table 2. Checklist of indicators of a balanced fertile menstrual cycle

A fertile balanced menstrual cycle is ideally:

- between 28 and 31 days long
- with menstruation lasting 4-5 days
- the blood is
  - neither too runny nor too sticky
  - deep red in colour, almost as if caused by a cut
  - without clots
  - without pain or spotting experienced at any part of the cycle
- the basal body temperature (BBT) should not waver for more than 0.1 degrees Celsius in each phase
  - with the BBT in the follicular phase hovering around 36.2-36.5°
  - rising up to 36.7-37.0° in the luteal phase
- ovulation should occur on day 12 or 13
  - with a thermal shift of 0.3-0.5° in 1-2 days
- cervical mucus is observed throughout the cycle
  - with runny, cloudy mucus during infertile days
  - with stretchy, clear mucus during fertile days around ovulation

Examples for infertile/imbalanced menstrual cycles are:

- dark purple coloured clotted menstrual blood linked with heavy flow and long cycles
- pink watery scanty flow of blood
- a slow rise of temperature/extended thermal shift of more than 2 days from follicular to luteal phase
- absence of fertile mucus

References: [15-19]

Figure 2A illustrates the BBT pattern of a balanced fertile menstrual cycle, and Table 2 provides a checklist of indicators of a balanced fertile menstrual cycle. The BBT should hover around 36.2-36.5 °C in the first part of the cycle, also known as the follicular phase, and between 36.7-37.0 °C in the second part of the cycle, known as the luteal phase. A balanced fertile cycle is 28-31 days long with ovulation occurring on day 12-13 indicated by a thermal shift of 0.3-0.5 °C (Fig 2A). The colour of the menstrual blood should have a deep red colour, as if caused by a cut, with no clots, and bleeding should last for 4-5 days. Menstrual flow should be moderate with no brown spotting. In a balanced menstrual cycle no pain or discomfort is felt during the cycle, before or during menstruation. A cervical mucus discharge is observed during the cycle, more runny and cloudy during infertile days, and stretchy and transparent like egg white during fertile days around ovulation (Table 2).

Variations of this menstrual pattern are indicators of imbalance and possible causes of compromised fertility (Table 1). Figures 2B-D illustrate three example of common TCM pattern in infertility.

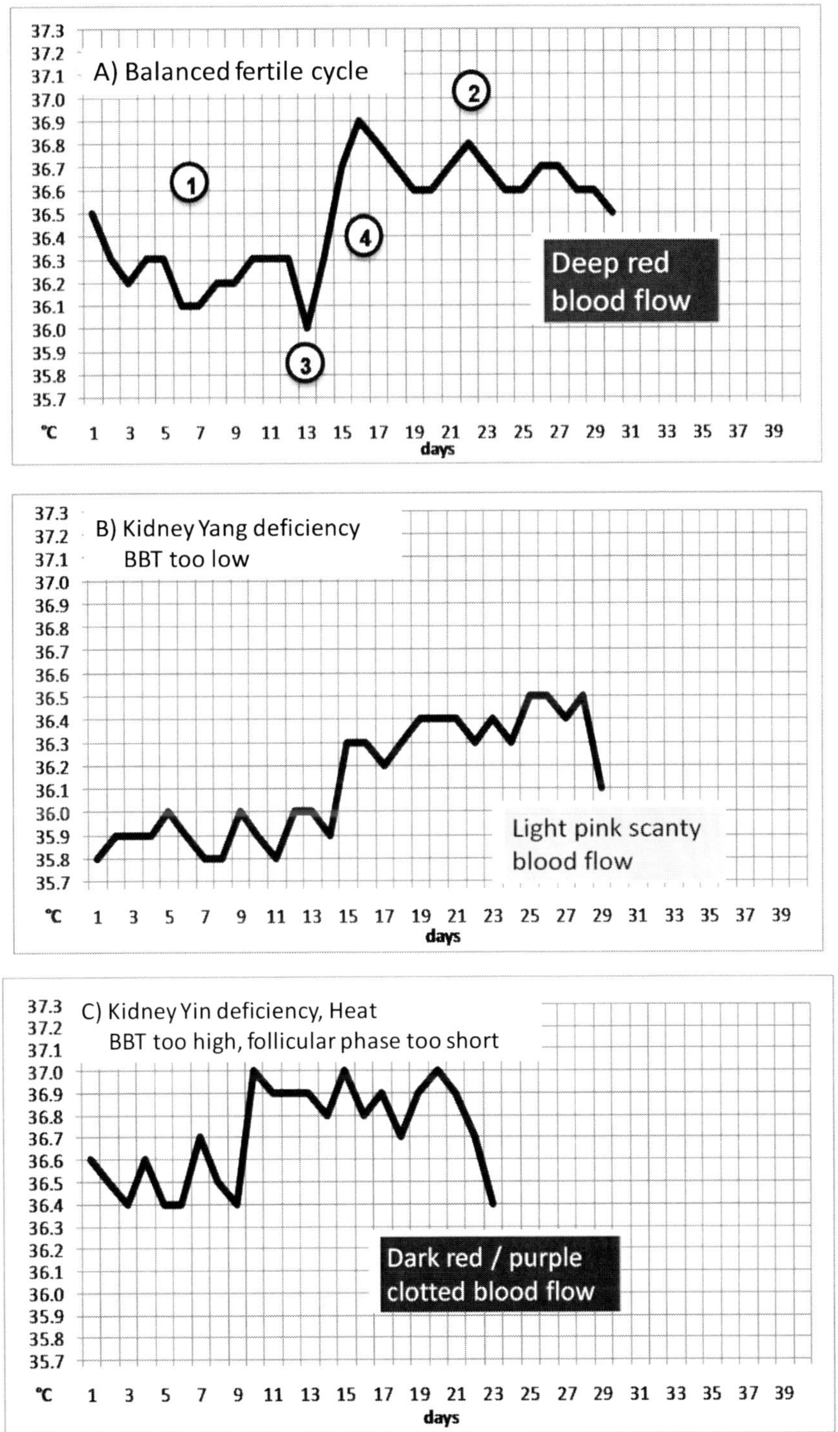

Figure 2. (Continued)

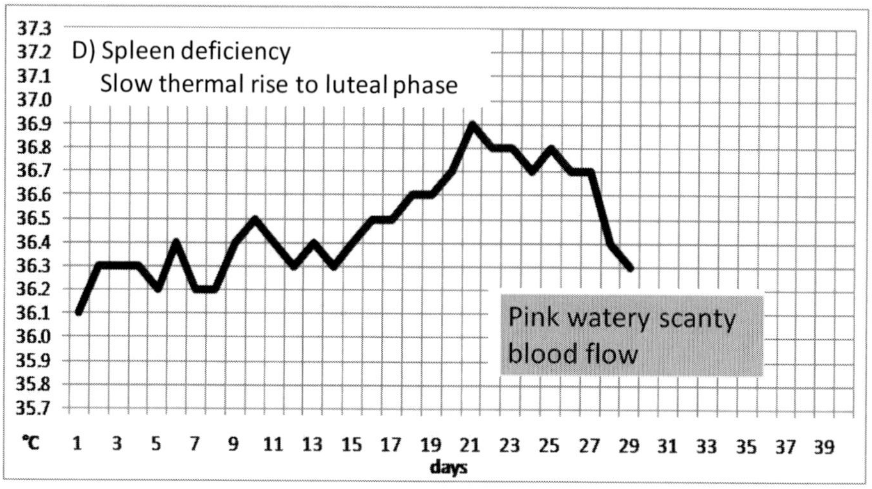

Figure 2. Figure 2A illustrates the basal body temperature (BBT) of a balanced fertile menstrual cycle, (1) follicular phase, (2) luteal phase, (3) ovulation, (4) thermal shift.

Figure 2B illustrates a low BBT, linked with light pink scanty blood flow, as well as a pale swollen tongue and a deep, slow, weak pulse, which is associated with the TCM pattern of Kidney Yang deficiency. Other common symptoms associated with Kidney Yang deficiency are pale complexion, fatigue, loose stools, feeling cold, low energy and low libido.

Figure 2C illustrates a high BBT and short follicular phase, linked with dark purple and often clotted blood, as well as a red, often peeled tongue with yellow coating and rapid, thin, wiry pulse, which is associated with Kidney Yin deficiency Heat. Other common symptoms associated with the TCM pattern of Kidney Yin deficiency Heat are red cheeks, hot sweaty palms/soles, hot flushes, insomnia, agitation, constipation, and thirst.

Figure 2D illustrates a slow thermal rise to the luteal phase spreading over more than 2 days, linked with pink watery scanty blood flow, as well as a swollen tongue with white fur, and a weak and slippery pulse, which is associated with the TCM pattern of Spleen deficiency. Other common symptoms associated with Spleen deficiency are a pale complexion, poor appetite, listlessness, and loose stools.

Discussion

Our meta-analyses of 8 RCTs and 7 cohort studies involving 1621 women with infertility suggest that the likelihood of achieving pregnancy with Chinese Herbal Medicine (CHM) are about three times greater than with conventional WM treatment using standard medication or IVF. Clinical pregnancy rates of about 60% were achieved with Chinese Herbal Medicine therapy over 4 months compared with 30% using WM fertility drug treatment, or IVF over 12 months.

Our findings were in line with results of a meta-analysis by See et al. (2011) comparing the effect of Traditional Chinese Herbal Medicine with Western Medical drug treatment using a different set of randomised controlled trials published in the Chinese literature compared with our meta-analysis of articles in English [20, 25]. The meta-analysis by See et al. (2011) including 13 RCTs and involving 1202 women reported a 2.6 higher likelihood of pregnancy with Chinese herbal medicine compared with Western medical drug therapy, and a mean pregnancy rate of 63% with CHM versus 39% with WM drug treatment [25].

Furthermore, we compared approaches to diagnosis and treatment of infertility of two different medical systems (TCM versus WM). While the approach to infertility treatment might differ between the TCM and WM model, the desired outcome in both is the achievement of a viable pregnancy. In TCM, the diagnostic and treatment approach to conditions such as PCOS and endometriosis is not any different than to amenorrhea, dysmenorrhea, irregular menses or unexplained infertility.

PCOS, for example, is one of the most common endocrine disorders affecting approximately 5-10% of women of reproductive age and is thought to be one of the leading causes of female subfertility [26]. PCOS is associated with amenorrhea or oligomenorrhea, irregular menses, hirsutism, obesity, insulin resistance, acne, hair loss, and infertility. The treatment of PCOS in the WM model involves prescription of the contraceptive pill, anti-diabetic drugs, gonadotropin (glycoprotein hormone), clomiphene (estrogen receptor modulator), sometimes surgery to destruct excess antral follicles, and IVF [26]. In contrast, TCM therapy uses herbal formulae or acupuncture treatment to restore, nourish, and resolve underlying imbalances associated with PCOS such as Kidney Jing deficiency, Phlegm-Damp accumulation, Liver Qi stagnation, Blood stasis, or Liver fire [14-16].

Additionally, 20-30% of women with fertility problems are diagnosed with endometriosis, which is associated with dispersed uterine tissue in the abdominal cavity causing inflammation and adhesions, and can lead to fallopian tube blockage, ovarian cysts and abdominal pain during bowel movements, urination, or sexual intercourse. Western Medical therapy can involve invasive laparoscopy and removal of excess tissue or cysts [27].

There is no word for 'endometriosis' in TCM classical texts [14, 28]. Instead, the clinical picture is described as dysmenorrhea or abdominal masses. TCM therapy involves the treatment of Liver Qi stagnation, Blood stasis, accumulation of Phlegm, and other potential underlying imbalances [14-16].

Women and couples experiencing infertility may benefit from a holistic approach, inclusion of the menstrual cycle as a diagnostic tool, and integration of therapies such as TCM to improve fertility and pregnancy outcomes, shorten treatment time frames, and reduce the emotional and financial burden.

In 2010, a 3-month treatment period with TCM including diagnosis, consultation, herbal formulae and acupuncture cost about $600-800 A$, whereas an IVF treatment cycle incurred an estimated fee of A$6,000-7,000 [29].Health fund rebates are available for TCM consultations and acupuncture, but not for herbal formulae [30]. TCM practice in Australia will become more transparent and consistent with the introduction of mandatory registration nationally in July 2012, as currently practiced in Victoria only [31].

Conclusion

Our meta-analyses suggest Traditional Chinese Herbal Medicine to be more effective in the treatment of female infertility achieving on average a 60% pregnancy rate over 4 months compared with 30% achieved with standard Western Medical drug treatment, or IVF over 12 months.

The TCM approach to infertility treatment integrates the menstrual cycle as a simple, non-invasive, sensitive, motivational, diagnostic tool to understanding a women's fertility status.

Our findings suggest that the integration of TCM diagnostic tools and therapy in the current WM model of infertility treatment could improve pregnancy rates while reducing treatment time frames and emotional and financial burden.

In this review we focused on the TCM approach to and diagnosis of infertility, a review of herbal formulae used in TCM therapy, and comparison of therapies combining TCM and ART/IVF were outside the scope of this review.

Parts 3 and 4:

Interviews with Women Seeking Holistic Therapies Including Traditional Chinese Medicine to Overcome Infertility

'I don't believe in unexplained'

Prologue

What do you do if you have been trying for a baby for a long time? You might have been to a fertility clinic and have had all the standard tests done, and nothing unusual indicated a cause for your infertility. You might have been told that your infertility is unexplained, and you should just keep trying. Even if you might have endured more invasive tests, perhaps had some surgery, but there's still no progress. Is in-vitro-fertilisation (IVF) the only option? Might there be another way of understanding your fertility? Can you personally improve your fertility? Can you take control? Is there hope?

This chapter is based on interviews with women who experienced infertility and who have sought a holistic approach in complementary therapies including naturopathy and Traditional Chinese Medicine (TCM). For our study, we recruited women with infertility, aged 20-45 years, Australia-wide between November 2008 and February 2010, through TCM practitioners, Internet forums, and newspaper advertisements [11].

The majority of women had postgraduate qualifications (76%) and were born in Australia (80%). Most women in our study had problems with conception (76%), and one-fifth had not been able to carry a pregnancy to term (24%). A number of women had secondary infertility. Two-thirds (68%) of women had attended a fertility clinic and then proceeded to TCM, of those 56% had been unsuccessful with IVF and sought other treatment options. Others (32%) chose to try TCM first.

Here they tell their stories.

Some women had problems conceiving, some had suffered miscarriages or stillbirths, most had been told that their infertility was 'unexplained'. Women share their journey of trying to achieve a viable pregnancy, some for as long as 10 years, what they did, how they felt, how they coped. They reveal where they found support, empowerment and importantly, hope.

All women agreed that awareness and recognition of holistic therapies such as Traditional Chinese Medicine (TCM) in relation to fertility is low, and wished to raise awareness and help other women by telling their story. Each of the women's stories is unique including the reasons for infertility, how they navigated the health system, what support they had and how they coped. Their stories display the diversity of infertility and treatment approaches, and shed light on relevant lifestyle and environmental factors, as well as menstrual health, often dismissed in a conventional medical diagnosis.

Information on TCM and fertility is sparse. Fertility specialists are often unaware of or reluctant to explore the causes of infertility using information the menstrual cycle has to offer.

Women's individual stories are told in their own voice, how women improved their fertility, overcame recurrent miscarriage, conception problems or secondary infertility. Women inform how a holistic approach can find underlying reasons for 'unexplained infertility'. They recollect how personalised care and continuity of care through a holistic health practitioner enabled better understanding and knowledge of fertility indicators, which in turn gave women hope, control and empowerment. They describe how the holistic approach explores and includes general health and wellbeing, nutrition and mind-body medicine on their path of overcoming infertility. All the women we interviewed emphasised the importance of balanced support, open-mindedness, persistence and self-believe.

These stories support a better understanding of the menstrual cycle - including changes in body temperature, mucus, pain and distension, and understanding of how lifestyle, diet and infection influence these menstrual patterns - can help women in general in their reproductive years, not only in relation to their fertility but also in relation to their general health and wellbeing.

Part 3: Listen to your Body

In part 3 of this chapter, four women tell their story of infertility, their experience with conventional medicine and holistic approaches, how they coped and what supported them. All learnt more about their menstrual cycle with the help of their holistic TCM practitioners, how the details of their menstrual cycle give clues on underlying fertility. It's not just about regularity, or the length of the cycle, as the first story illustrates, but also about the quality of the menstrual blood, the basal body temperature pattern, and – let's not forgot – the mucus or discharge pattern between bleeds. All women wished they had known more about these fertility indicators before they embarked on the journey of trying for a baby.

Story 1: A Fertile Menstrual Cycle

Jules has been trying to conceive for about five years. Her fertility specialist treated her endometriosis, and put her on fertility hormones, but could do no more. Then, a friend of Jules told her about a TCM practitioner.

Menstrual Cycle

I wasn't regular until I went on the pill at about 16. I was also a very heavy bleeder with clots, like skin. But that all stopped when I went on the pill and I was on that for a good 10 years. I'm 35 now and I came off the pill a few years ago. That's a long time.

Trying to Conceive

Amazingly enough I thought I'd become irregular after I came off the pill, but I remained regular to the dot every month. I was off the pill for about a year and I hadn't got pregnant and I didn't think it would take that long. That's when I went to see a fertility specialist who was referred by my GP. I was put on Clomid (Clomiphene, an estrogen receptor modulator) for about three months before I had laparoscopy. This found that I had endometriosis, which I was very surprised because I had no pain and they also found two large cysts on each ovary. The obstetrician said that there was no way I would conceive with these conditions. So he operated and fixed all that and then he put me on Clomid for a further six months, but still nothing. He said, "I can't really do much more for you".

I don't drink and I don't smoke. I'm relatively healthy and I'm very fit but sometimes I wonder if part of the problem is that I work so hard on our farm and we are always tired. We're so tired all the time. I have talked to the specialist about that though and he said for me the Clomid should be overriding that. If I am tired he said I should be fine. So then I think, "well I'm quite healthy so what's wrong with me?

My TCM Experience

During that last six months a friend of mine told me how her daughter had endometriosis and had trouble conceiving and she went to see a TCM practitioner after being told that she wouldn't be able to have children. She ended up having three children. I've always known about Chinese medicine, but never thought I needed it. What would I need it for? I was fine half the year. So, it wasn't till I actually started thinking that something was wrong and that I wanted to get it sorted out. I thought, "I want to try." If other people have had success seeing this TCM practitioner, maybe I will too. The thing with IVF is that so many people miscarry anyway because their eggs or endometrium aren't any good. I figured that if I can get my body right it's only going to help. It's too early for me to think about IVF because I'm still learning so much. So I went and the TCM practitioner had me on herbal tea and told me what I should and shouldn't eat, which I'm trying very hard to follow. I am not supposed to eat any carbohydrates at all. So no bread, rice, pumpkin, sugar or alcohol. She said I shouldn't have juice either. She gave me a book of things I should and shouldn't eat, but I don't do it 100 per cent. I'm trying really, really hard though.

The TCM practitioner said that I had toxins, and that would be what caused the endometriosis because the body is not working properly. She's trying to flush the toxins out with the blood type diet. She did a blood test and then told me what I should be eating according to that. She is very positive. She says "it's going to happen" and is very supportive. She tells me that it's on me if I don't do the right thing by not eating what she tells me to eat and not drinking the tea, then I'm just delaying it myself. She's brilliant for the fact that I could see a difference from when I first started seeing her. My husband recently injured himself and I couldn't see the TCM practitioner for a few months and I couldn't get any tea. I went off the tea for a couple of weeks and straight away I got pimples, my temperature went up and I thought, "wow, the tea is obviously making a difference!" I'm actually taking more interest in doing my charts every day also. I had never known about the significance of your body's temperature until the TCM practitioner showed me where my temperature should be, and then I looked at mine and thought, oh that's not right, is it? I had no idea. It was not until she told me about it. I'm paying a little bit more attention to myself and I probably wouldn't have before. Everybody always said, "you're ovulating when you see mucus like eggwhite", and I just thought, "I don't know what you're talking about. I don't see that". Even now filling these charts in, I do find it difficult because it asks me questions and I think, "I don't see that, I don't know that". So I'm probably not as observant as I should be but I definitely now know more about making babies.

I didn't realise that Chinese medicine includes your diet and how much of a difference that can make. I've learned a lot about that and I have noticed that since I've been taking the herbal tea and since I've been cutting down on carbs, my discharge has changed. *Everyone always used to say that when you're ovulating you'll know, but I didn't because I haven't had any mucus. So that has definitely changed. I don't have that sticky mucus but I have some discharge, whereas I didn't have any before, so now I'm looking at the pattern. And the temperature has changed. My temperature has dropped. When I first started seeing her I was always in the 36.6, 36.7, in the first phase I've definitely dropped, but not quite as much as she'd like me to drop.*

You wouldn't believe it. People tell you not to eat certain foods because they're bad and you think, "oh yeah, everything's bad", but it's not until you start doing what my TCM practitioner said that you believe it. I've cut sugar and I was very into sugar. I've cut it by about 85 per cent, which actually did make a difference and I lost weight. I probably lost about three kilos. She also looks at my husband and she's got him on a blood type diet as well. She explains that it's not all just about me. Even though we had his sperm tested and that was fine, she said that if he's tired or if he's lazy, then his sperm is going to come out quite lazy too. So she's helping us both. He had a different blood group to me and so he's meant to eat different things to me. He's actually allowed to have carbs. He doesn't eat them though, he won't do it because he feels bad for me. So he just goes without having any. He's allowed soft drink, but he won't. Plus I won't cook two separate meals. Every now and then I'll put potato in for him.

The TCM practitioner does say that this way of eating does not have to be for forever, it's just while I'm detoxing. Once I've done the detox I can have sugar but just not to the excess I used to have it. I always knew that I consumed too much sugar because I'd been to a GP once a long time ago for a normal check up and she actually said to me that I was hyperglycaemic and told me to cut back on sugar. That time I just ignored her because I didn't feel like it was doing anything to me. I thought that I was not sick and that I was okay. I had a few pimples which is what she obviously spotted, but I thought "who cares." Now I have learnt the impact it had. It obviously was doing something inside which was causing endometriosis, and maybe had I listened to the GP back then I wouldn't have had such a severe case of endometriosis. She didn't explain what it might be doing to my body.

I went back to the specialist recently and he basically said there's not much more that he can do, so I'm sticking with TCM for now. I'm very lucky I found out about my TCM practitioner because not only will she hopefully help me have a baby, she'll help me get myself sorted. I've also told all my family because it's not just about trying to have a baby, it's about your health. Everybody needs it.

I would hope that somehow TCM becomes better known because there'd be a lot of young women like me that are trying and never find out about someone like my TCM practitioner. They go to see a fertility specialist and then they go on IVF, probably have multiple cycles. I heard of someone who just did it for 10 years!

When my specialist said to me, "I can't help you anymore, but your options are IVF or adoption", it would have been lovely if he'd said, "your options are IVF, adoption, or you could try alternate therapy". Wouldn't it be nice. But that option is not given. Lucky for me I knew, but what about all the other poor women that don't know?

Coping Emotionally

I think I've been pretty good emotionally because I've actually had other friends who've had children and been trying for another one, and they've been in tears. I'm not at that stage. When I get my period I think, "oh great, here we go again". I get down, but not for long. I still think it's going to happen, so I'm not at that point where I'm depressed, miserable or sad. Everybody else thinks that I am stressed. Everybody tells me that I talk about it too much and worry about it too much that it's not going to happen because it's on my mind. But how could you get it off your mind? If you're trying to do something, how can it not be on your mind? But why should I not use my support group and use any help that I can get? If I had to go through it and keep it to myself, it might upset me because sometimes I need to vent. So I talk to people, my sister or friends, and in my community we all get close and we all talk. It makes me feel better. They give me support and sometimes I just want to hear that.

There are times when you need to talk and there are times you get a little down and it would be very hard for women out there to have no one. I must say that my TCM practitioner is very good for that. She's very good to just explain and tell you how it is whilst being so positive. Even if you go there feeling a little bit negative, she's so positive and I think, I can do this.

I talk to my husband all the time. He knows more than anyone because he lets me talk about it. He doesn't judge me or tell me I'm worrying too much, so he's the best one for me to talk to. He's very good. I'd be lost without him. I'm from an ethnic family and so mum's not good at talking about illness and womanly things. Mum will just tell me that I worry too much so we don't talk about it. She's good, she's always been there for me and she'll always help me if I need help, but she's just thinks that there's nothing wrong with me and doesn't believe that I need to see anyone. "You're just fine, it'll happen so get over it".

The Difference between TCM and Western Practitioners

Both my TCM practitioner and Western doctor are both lovely, but both very different. My TCM practitioner explains things while my specialist only tells me what's wrong. "Okay, you've got endometriosis, here're some photos. I'll cut it out and you'll be right now". He has actually told me test results that I still don't understand. Half the time when I go there I'm so dumbfounded and nervous and I don't ask what I should ask. However, I feel like I can ask my TCM practitioner more and she explains to me what is happening and how to prevent it from coming back. Maybe it's because she is a female, but both are very nice and happy to help and happy to answer any questions. My specialist actually knows I have been seeing a TCM practitioner, and he was fine. He said that I should try anything.

I haven't told my gynaecologist about the changes I've experiencing with my cycle since I've been seeing the TCM practitioner. It's awful but he doesn't ask how long I menstruate for. He doesn't ask about discharge or anything like that. He doesn't ask, he just says that as long as I have sex every second day from day X to day Y, I'm covered". He doesn't acknowledge my cycle much. So he's not taking any notice of what my body is telling me. Not at all. He just tells me what a normal person's cycle does. Let's say you're abnormal. To cover it I want you to start from here and finish here". But he's done my ovulation as every month I had to go for blood tests to see how I was ovulating. I think he's medically done everything that he can do. I'm taking advice from both. Do a little bit from him and with my TCM practitioner I'm fixing my diet.

Certainly when I first went to my GP the first time and said I was trying to conceive, it would have been really handy if I'd been given a couple of warnings such as, do you know what to look for? Do you know about the temperature? Do you know about the discharge? That would have been handy because then I would have paid more attention at that point.

Story 2: Overcoming Recurrent Miscarriages

The next story highlights that even if conception is not the problem, recurrent miscarriages are a sign for a non-ideal environment to maintain a healthy pregnancy. A Chinese proverb says "Cultivate the soil before planting the seed". Related to fertility, the seed are the eggs and sperm, while the soil is the body's environment, which includes the women's endometrium, the lining of the uterus where the fertilised egg implants.

Rachel had tried for about three years to have a baby. While she easily conceived, she suffered multiple miscarriages.

Conceiving Was Never a Problem

I got married when I was 27 and I thought we'd see how I'd go getting pregnant. I went off the pill and the next month I was pregnant. We weren't trying very hard so to speak. That shocked me because normally it takes a while for the pill to get out of your system. I had been taking it straight for seven years without any breaks. We lost that first one. It was around 11 weeks but the foetus had not even made it to 6 or 7 weeks. We tried again, and got pregnant not long after. We lost that one also, around the same time. We went for a scan but there was no heartbeat, maybe that was the third one.

I had no problems at all falling pregnant and it was probably every three to four months that I was pregnant. I would find out that I was pregnant, loose it after a couple of months, then have a month or two break to get my cycle back into order and so then it's probably every four to five months that I would get pregnant again.

I went to see a specialist at the recurrent miscarriage clinic and he ran the normal standard genetics test to see if there was anything standing out with myself and my husband. That all came back fine and they just said "that's the way it is, everything's fine, it's nature, maybe there was something wrong with the baby." The specialist can't find any reason for it, we have no reason. They tried to be helpful but they couldn't, they didn't have anything to give me.

There were four miscarriages by that stage. I was told that it's one in every four pregnancies that miscarry. It was pretty specific, and I was four in four so I just thought it's ridiculous, it's no longer natural. It was hard because obviously there was something wrong.

My TCM Experience

A girlfriend of mine had been going to a Chinese herbalist. When I first heard about it from her I thought that it makes sense because Chinese have been using these medicines for thousands of years and it works for them, maybe I'll give it a go. It was starting to get a bit much and when I first saw the Chinese herbalist, it was very scary, because if that wasn't going to work, what would happen then? Then I would have had to look at all the other options. I didn't want to have to do anything that hurt.

I didn't ask the TCM practitioner too many questions but I did ask whether there was a reason for my recurrent miscarriages. She explained that I had a weakened Qi (life energy), and my body is very hot and it needed to be cooled down. My body was not conducive to having a child because it was so hot and my body wasn't putting as much nutrients into my blood as it could be. It makes sense to say that I'm too hot, because I walk around in t-shirts.

The TCM practitioner's qualifications were up on her wall and I've read them many times. She's got certificates to practise herbal medicine. They were all very qualified, she and her acupuncturist. It was like going to the doctor's surgery. Instead of a Bachelor of Surgery, they've got their equivalent in Chinese Medicine.

I'd heard about Traditional Chinese Medicine before, but I hadn't put any weight on it. It wasn't something I would have thought of doing. When people think they can't get pregnant they usually go to IVF or they sometimes try natural herbs. I never see anything on TV for Chinese herbalists and I haven't seen any adverts anywhere for my herbalist's business. They've got little brochures in the waiting room on Chinese herbs and infertility or endometriosis and other conditions. It's not advertising themselves so much, it's just saying Chinese herbs might be able to help with these conditions. I had no idea what I was in for with the sticks and the herbs. It was like twigs and bark. Most of the time we took the herbs and cooked those up. They became liquid, it was dirty mud water. Not very pleasant to take. I think the herbs were the main medicine. The acupuncture was complementary, just to ensure that we were doing it all right. I wasn't a big fan of acupuncture. It stings more when you get the ones that make your legs jump (electro-acupuncture). My acupuncturist said that in China they want to feel that so then they know that it's working. It wasn't something that I found relaxing. Once he put the needles in it was fine but the whole thing just stressed me a little bit so I just did it on a needs basis. I had it with the second baby to prepare me for birth. I thought about it with my first son, but didn't have it. I'm sure if I needed to I would be happy to go back. I've got no problem, if there's something that I think TCM could help me with I would try them.

In the TCM clinic I was treated with a more holistic feel, looking at everything that's happening in my body rather than just the reproductive aspects or the genetics. I was given herbs and acupuncture for six months before the next pregnancy and this one stuck. I had a son. He's going to be 3 in May. When I went and saw the specialist in the recurrent miscarriage clinic when I was pregnant, he didn't ask anything about what I had been doing. I told him that I'd actually gone and seen a Chinese herbalist but Western medicine doesn't give any credit to them at all.

We left it for a while, and when he was about one year old I fell pregnant again. This time the doctors had all told me that I would be fine because my body knows what to do. I was hoping that's what would happen but I lost that one. Again, I thought it was ridiculous. So I went and saw my herbalist and acupuncturist three months before I wanted to fall pregnant again and lo and behold this one stuck as well. This is pregnancy two and both those pregnancies have been when I've seen a herbalist and acupuncturist.

The evidence is overwhelming and whenever I've spoken to someone who says they've lost some children, I tell them to try this.

After seven pregnancies and the only two that have stuck were when I've used these TCM therapies. I think it's a bit more than coincidence.

If I wanted another child, I wouldn't want to fluke it. It would need to be planned and I would go back to the TCM practitioner again.

Coping with the Emotions

After the first couple of miscarriages I just said "well these things happen". It's a bit of a shame, maybe there was something wrong with the foetuses. But as it went on it was hard when there was nothing I could do. Why was this happening? I'm healthy, I'm young, it doesn't make any sense. I was stubborn more than anything else. I said to myself "I'm going to have a baby, how are we going to do this", and like anyone you do what you need to do to get through. I'm not very good at asking other people for things, so it was mainly me and my husband. He was just stoic and kept telling me that it was all right and that it'll happen. He was very supportive, I don't know how it affected him, and I think it did of course, but he was much better supporting me than breaking down. Also some of the forums on the Internet helped me cope. It was good to read that other people were having the same problems. Once I found the Huggies website, I realised it encompassed everything and that's interesting knowing that other people were in similar positions.

Raising Awareness

Where I live we have a newspaper 'CITY Child' and it's got really good articles about mums and health. It also has advertisements for places to have parties and other entertainment. There is also a wanted section for people looking for egg donors and sperm donors, so it's all around people wanting to be pregnant and have children. I think CITY Child would be a good place to advertise TCM, because if it's on TV or radio advertising then I would not give much credit to it. I would think it would sound like a scam and not sound reliable. Whereas if CITY Child had a half page advert, explaining TCM, that to me would give it more credit. It would almost be like word of mouth and word of mouth works for me.

People shouldn't have to go through recurrent miscarriages without knowing about TCM therapy. Then they can make a choice, they can try TCM, they don't have to but at least they know about it.

Story 3: Overcoming Conception Problems

The next story highlights that a healthy body needs a healthy mind. Danny tried for six years to fall pregnant before discovering meditative practice and alternative holistic therapies including Chinese Medicine. Believe in herself, an open mind and persistence led her on the path to overcoming infertility. She is mum to a little boy and baby twins.

Success

You've got to be very careful what you wish for [laughs]. We tried for six years to have a child and nothing was happening. We'd had unprotected sex for six years and you would think after that time you would have nailed it once. Finally I gave birth to Sam and then 18 months later we had twins. The twins just turned three and they're so full on and boisterous. It's weird that you wish for that for so long and you want it and now you've got it.

Trying to Conceive

I had IVF twice, in two different clinics, and we never really got off the ground with it because I always had in the back of my head that I didn't need it. I wasn't upset about it. There was never any time where I thought that it was never going to happen but then as the time got longer I thought that we should look into it a bit more. I think it's sad that the first reaction is to go and see a doctor and go to IVF because maybe if my first reaction had been to go and see a naturopath, things might have happened a lot quicker for me. It's just how you're brought up, to go see a doctor and that they'll fix it. They'll give you a tablet and you'll be fine. But I would not have gone down the IVF path, if I had known what I know now.

I was injecting all these chemicals but I was thinking it wasn't right, something's not right here. It wasn't long before we walked away thinking the obstetrician obviously got to meet his quota of successes to be funded again the following year and if I looked like I wasn't going to be one of those success stories then it might be better for him to cut his ties with me. ***The obstetrician said to me, "look just forget it, it's not going to happen." "It's never going to happen, go buy a puppy or you might want to look at a surrogate."*** *I walked out of there. He had said it was unexplained infertility, or maybe I was going through an early menopause. This did make sense because my mum did but not until she was into her 40s and I was 36.*

The disappointing thing was when I walked out of the doctor's office and he said that he had a counsellor that I could go and see. But when I walked into the counsellor's office, she had nothing, no other alternatives to offer me. I was expecting for her to tell me that she had a list of naturopaths I could go to or that I should try yoga and meditation. I thought there would be other alternative options, but they had nothing. She was more of a grief counsellor to helping me get over the fact that it was never going to happen. I walked out of there feeling really angry that there was nowhere else to go and that I had to work all that out for myself. If I wasn't switched on, if I wasn't too bright then I would not have done anything about it. Then you'd spend the rest of your life so bitterly disappointed that you were never able to have children.

Turning Point - Believe in Oneself

I just couldn't believe that as a female you were put on this earth for the one job that you were meant to do and I couldn't do it. That wasn't me, because I can do everything. I had that running over and over in my head. Fair enough you can't dance or you can't cook or you can't sew, but to not be able to have a child! I just couldn't fathom that at all and I'd always been really fit and healthy so it's got to work.

I've always been very confident, over confident and always been able to achieve whatever I've put my mind to and I'm very competitive. Like Mum, she especially was competitive and whatever you wanted you'd get because you'd work hard and whatever had to be done.

Trying Alternative Therapies

I started to get into yoga and so I was open to all the different types of alternative therapies that were out there. Through that whole journey of yoga I came into contact with so many different people with different views on how the universe operates that you start to open up more to different options. The yoga school I went to was into active births, home births, so the teacher was right into fertility. My girlfriend and I found a yoga class and that is where it all started for me because we did our class, our stretches and at the end of the class our teacher would do meditation/relaxation and would always ask us to put ourselves in our favourite place and whatever's missing in that favourite place, add that thing. Always have that in your mind. She had no idea what I was trying to do and every week I thought that the only thing missing is a baby on a rug laying there kicking while I'm doing my yoga in our backyard. So I always had that affirmation and I just kept that strong in my mind. It amazed me how powerful it is. I got friends that are open to that sort of thing and then other friends thought I was a bit of a irrational. But I just kept pushing through with that and I think that had a lot to do with my success.

Then I went through the whole stage of just clearing out my life. We ran our own business, and I told my husband that it was stressing me out. I told him that we were going to get someone in to do some of my work. So then I started more yoga and was also referred by a friend to a naturopath who was really good. He was so gentle and lovely and he just listened to me. We talked about what I was doing in my life at the time and what we can clear out. Many people that I came in touch with at that time were all about getting rid of things in my head to make room for something to come, for the baby to come. It was a clearing out process, "go home and get rid of all your rubbish".

I had a couple of reflexology sessions. When I had my little boy the reflexologist came to the hospital to see me. "See what I did!" It's hard to pinpoint which therapy can be accounted for. It might have been the Bowen therapy, it might have been the reflexology or it might have been the fact that I was in a completely different state of mind after doing yoga every day for so long. But with the Chinese herbs I could see a difference in my menstrual cycle.

My TCM Experience

The naturopath recommended a Chinese herbalist who was a little Chinese man not far from where I live. I went to his house and I could hardly understand him but we had so much fun trying to understand each other. I'd just sit down and he would put his hand on my pulse and he was feeling for my Qi (life energy), for the flow of my Qi. I thought it felt a little weird but I was happy to do whatever it took, I would have done anything. He would tell me what I was stressing about, and was actually really specific. "You're really stressing over the fact that you can't have this baby and it's really affecting your day-to-day life and you need to start clearing your head." I told me I was too much of a thinker, which I agreed. I do stress over trivial things. Every time I went in there he said I had to clear my mind and not to fill my head with trivial, insignificant worries that are going to bog me down because I need to make way for the baby to come.

His main diagnosis was that my menstruation cycle had been out of balance for so long, because of what we eat, the way we live our lives and the stress that we're putting on our bodies and minds.

I had been on the pill when I was 18 and I didn't come off that until I was about 30 so that was a long time on the pill - as the Chinese herbalist explained - had stuffed my whole body around in the first place.

I was amazed how little I knew about my body and when I started plotting my period and my menstrual cycle I thought, "I don't know anything about this, I've never bothered to pay any attention to it." But then I think it's like anything, you don't know about something until you start to do the research and start to learn about it.

I always had irregular periods that were all over the place. They were spasmodically, not every month but every now and then. Also the eggs that I was producing were not of good quality and my husband had a low sperm count. He was a smoker which probably didn't help, but he'd already had a child and so he'd proved his point.

The TCM practitioner used herbs as a way of clearing and restoring that Qi, restoring the balance. Once you can do that internally with the herbs and get your mind clear and head towards the thing that you want to achieve, then you've got more of a chance of getting there, if everything's in balance. I told him all that stuff about the endometriosis and the egg quality but I don't think he was that interested in that. I think his theory was more that the herbs will put everything in balance and then all those things that are wrong will get right by themselves because you've put yourself back into balance.

He seemed to hit it on the head but again you're clutching at straws. He'd go off into his kitchen and to me it was like he walked out into his backyard and just scooped up all the dirt, leaves, mud, stones, bricks and whatever he could find and put it in a bag and said, "there you go, go home, cook that and drink it." I don't know what was in it but I was just happy to do anything. He was just really lovely. He could have been giving me bark chips for all I knew. I didn't know and I didn't care.

There was a change in my menstrual cycle, definitely. I'm definite that Chinese herbs made it spot on, exact to the day and changed the texture, colour and look of my blood. I could see a difference in my menstrual cycle and the way I was bleeding and I was spot on because I'd never been regular in my life with my menstrual cycle and all of a sudden I'm spot on to the day and it was a different colour. So you could actually see, that was real evidence for me that the Chinese herbs were working.

Finding out I Was Pregnant

I had been plotting my cycle for a while, also looking at mucus and temperature. I would have been on the herbs for about six months when I got pregnant. Before I knew I was pregnant, I actually went to my second IVF clinic because I'd got to the point where I was doing all the alternative stuff and I thought I was ready to try again. A lady started doing all the tests. She did a saline sonogram but said that she couldn't get the saline to stick and that she would do some more tests and ring me with the results. I was heading back home when she rang me and told me that I had better pull off the road. I thought, "here we go, I've heard this story a hundred times". I was starting to become disappointed because the only news I'd ever had was, "no there's no other tests and no you're not pregnant". So I pulled over and she said, "I worked out why the test wouldn't work. It's because you're already pregnant." I had myself in that frame of mind that I was ready for disappointment and so when I hung up and drove off I thought, "what a mean thing to ring me and tell me that I'm pregnant when I'm not". So even though I really wanted to be pregnant I also had it in my head that maybe it was never going to happen. Then as I kept driving to meet with my husband, it slowly started to dawn on me that it's finally happened.

When I got pregnant, my girlfriend, a midwife and she had suggested a woman obstetrician that all the midwives go to. I thought there's no higher recommendation. I went to her and her medical partner was my previous obstetrician. When I walked into her office he asked what I was doing there. I told him that I was pregnant and he said "no way," he wouldn't and couldn't believe it. Then when I was having my consultation with her he knocked on the door and asked her to confirm that I was actually pregnant. He said it was a miracle. Then 18 months later I was back in there saying, "guess what, I'm having twins". But he didn't want to know how it happened. He was completely closed to the fact that it had anything to do with the Chinese herbs. Six months after I had the twins, my female obstetrician sent me an email and asked for information on the naturopath and Chinese herbalist I saw so she could pass it on to another patient of hers. She was somewhat open to it in the end but during the process she wouldn't have a bar of it. I would ask her, "how can you not?" and she said, "it was a fluke". We had lots of discussions about it though and I asked her why she wouldn't rather send someone out to give them hope." Her answer was that she wouldn't want someone to agonise over something that they're probably not going to have." I felt that it's not just giving them something to hang on to but you've also sent someone out there who's chosen a healthier lifestyle.

Doctors' Influence and Responsibility

There was a girl that worked in my office at the time and she'd given up trying to get pregnant because her obstetrician had also told her that it was never going to happen. We have often talked about the fact that we both could have walked out of that office and just thought that was the end of it and just never tried again. But I walked out of there thinking, "no, that can't be right, there's got to be other ways". There's a real responsibility for doctors like that to be more open. How good would it have been if I could have walked out of my first obstetrician's office and have him recommend me to pop in next door and make an appointment with the naturopath and then that naturopath would have had his Chinese herbalist, his yoga rooms and his Bowen therapist or reflexologist. I got really angry and disappointed that the professionals weren't more open minded to alternatives because for me I really think that apart from the use of the Chinese herbs, it was very psychological because I'd got to the point where I was so ticked off that this wasn't going to happen that there had to be something to do. There had to be another alternative and there literally was nowhere for me to go from there. It wasn't until you start getting into that circle of yoga teachers and naturopaths that they start referring you.

My Second Pregnancy with Twins

At my 40th birthday I was giving a speech and saying, "guess what, I'm not drinking tonight and I feel really sick because I'm pregnant with twins". All my friends were gobsmacked. I can remember saying to my husband that if it took us six years to conceive our first child, it might take us a while to get pregnant again and so maybe we should try again as soon as we can.

It was a normal multiple births pregnancy, which is a lot different to a single pregnancy. It was all fine, everything was healthy. I carried them to nearly 39 weeks. That last trimester was just terrible. I was too big and I couldn't stand up half the time. Someone had to come and help me off the couch and when they were born they were both nearly 8 pound each. They were huge.

Story 4: Overcoming Secondary Infertility

Monique experienced secondary infertility. While she is a mum of two children (four and a half and three years of age), she had been trying for a third baby for a number of years unsuccessfully. Monique explains how she decided for TCM instead of IVF, and learnt that the right diet for her improved her fertility, visible through desired changes in her menstrual cycle. A few months after Monique told her story,TCM therapy has helped Monique fulfill her dream.

My First Two Children

I've got two children but I've been trying for a couple of years for a third. I always had very regular periods, about 28 to 30 day cycles and I knew when I ovulated because I had pain in my side and all the usual signs. There were no problems at all and we had decided we'd have children. I hadn't taken the pill for years and we got pregnant with our first child without really trying. I had been on the pill for three to four years but after I got married I stopped taking it as I didn't particularly like it. We were just careful to avoid times of the month but when I fell pregnant we were so happy that it happened.

When my son was about one and a half years old we decided to have another child. It took about three months for me to get pregnant and there were no problems. I breastfed for about nine months.

Trying to Conceive for the Third Time

We now had two boys and I suppose it was always in the back of my mind we would have liked another one. When my second son was about one and a half, we both thought another one would be okay so we tried and tried but my periods had been quite erratic since my second birth.

I went to my obstetrician and told him that I was having this strange bleeding between periods and then I'll get my period. There was lots of erratic bleeding with no sign of ovulation and no pain. It was very difficult to work out what was going on. He said, "Oh you're still breastfeeding, you've got to give yourself time." So we left it for quite a while after I had stopped breastfeeding and I went back to my GP and told her that we'd been trying and nothing had happened.

My obstetrician did an ultrasound and said that I had polycystic ovaries. I'd never had any indication of that before but I was a little bit overweight from the two pregnancies. He suggested that I go on Clomid (Clomiphene, an estrogen receptor modulator) to make me ovulate regularly and increase my chances of pregnancy. So I took Clomid for a few months on again, off again because it gave me headaches and I didn't feel 100% taking it.

My Experience with Naturopathy

At this time, a friend of mine had just finished her studies in naturopathy and some Chinese Medicine. Because she was just newly trained I went and saw her because it wasn't expensive. I didn't have to pay for the consult, I only had to pay for the herbs. I'm not sure if it is connected but I had seen her for about three months and had been taking herbs - that were in a liquid form - and then I got pregnant.

I told the gynaecologist about it and he said, "Look you may as well drink toilet water." That just made me feel ..., well maybe it is a load of hogwash. Especially because I was so Western medically orientated.

Miscarriage

At about 9 to 10 weeks of the pregnancy I had a miscarriage. I'd had a lot of bleeding during the pregnancy and it didn't feel the same as the others and I had no morning sickness.

The obstetrician said there were two reasons to have a miscarriage: one is genetic problems and the other is placenta problems. Because there was a lot of bleeding during the nine weeks, the egg hadn't attached properly from the start and the placenta hadn't grown properly. I had a D&C (dilation & curette) in the end because I had some bleeding but when it stopped, nothing happened for about four days and I was waiting and waiting but nothing happened. I initially thought I'd just leave it to happen naturally but then I felt I just can't get on with things if it's not finalised.

IVF or Not?

I went back on the Clomid for a few months but nothing happened. I went and saw the fertility specialist and I discussed the situation again with him. He said my only other option is to go to IVF. My husband and I have had long talks about IVF. Early in the year I was thinking I should just do it, but then I started thinking how it may not work anyway and financially it's a big cost, especially when we've already got two children. So we had long discussions about it and decided that we would just stick with the Clomid. But nothing happened.

It has been helpful to talk to other women about what I'm going through. There are lots of women who go through the same things. A friend of mine who's had IVF and has just had her second child is giving a strong push towards IVF. It's just that accepted form of treatment that people think that if you don't have success falling pregnant then you automatically will go. This is mainly from women who've had IVF. I haven't found that many women actually know about TCM or alternative ways, only a few. Some people really believe in it and some people think maybe it's a bit of hogwash. My husband is not particularly keen on IVF. He doesn't even like the idea of the Clomid. He *worries about the affect of those artificial hormones on your body and what affect it may have in 10 years' time. So he's not keen at all on doing things artificially basically. It doesn't thrill me to think about all the invasive things that you do to have IVF. I've spoken to a few people and I've looked IVF up on the internet so I basically know what they do. I think it's an emotional roller coaster. My obstetrician said it's up to me but it is a very emotionally traumatic time, because it may not work anyway. I feel with the way that my body has been that it probably wouldn't work because* ***it's not necessarily having an egg implanted, it's what comes after that. Keeping it there.*** *I don't know if I could cope with knowing that you've gone through all that and it hadn't worked.*

My obstetrician said 'look you can go to the IVF clinic and you can talk to them and they will say, "we can help you, we can, you've got 80% chance", but he said at the end of day it may not and he also says you're coming up to 38 and years go past and he was quite realistic about it.

The Idea of Traditional Chinese Medicine

A couple of years ago a friend had told me that she had lots of problems falling pregnant and she went to a Chinese herbalist. She said, "I can recommend her, she's really good." It had resulted in her having three children and even now she regularly goes back if she wants to loose a bit of weight or if she feels a bit flat. This was years ago that she had told me about it and three times I rang up and booked in but then cancelled at the last minute. I don't know whether I just thought it was a waste of time or I just wasn't ready to change my lifestyle and diet. I'm a trained nurse and it's so drummed into you that medicine is the best way and that Western Medicine is the only way I guess.

I started to feel well this year. I'm 38 and getting a bit older and if it hasn't worked now, maybe it won't ever work and maybe I should try TCM. I thought it would be the last thing I would try and see if that worked.

So on the fourth occasion I kept my appointment. I finally went and saw the TCM practitioner and now have been seeing her for almost 2 months. The TCM practitioner was very promising. ***She said that polycystic ovary syndrome is a Western disease and is a diet related thing that should not happen. She told me it was my lifestyle and what I'm eating is what is causing it.*** *She said these things don't happen in Chinese medicine. I think that because I'm 38 now my time is running out whereas she says, "You're not 45, you're only 38".*

My TCM Experience

When I go and see the TCM practitioner and tell her about what's happening, she's very good. She explains everything. Compared to conventional Western medical practitioner, she looks more at your whole body. She checks my pulse and looks at my tongue and she's not overly interested in one specific area.

She said that from the last two pregnancies my pancreas is very stressed and producing too much insulin. Then eating carbohydrates such as bread, cereal and fruit are making me produce a lot of insulin and that fluctuation of insulin affects my progesterone. If my insulin is high, my progesterone is low and also my temperature is very erratic and it is hard to maintain a pregnancy when your progesterone is low and your temperature is not regular.

The TCM practitioner put me on a strict diet and she gave me herbs. Each time I see her I ask questions so that I don't feel overwhelmed. She looks at my blood type and puts me on a diet in relation to what blood type I am. There are books about that. I am not allowed to eat any carbohydrates at all. No rice, pasta, bread. No fruit. No alcohol, tea or coffee. Green tea I can have. She said that when I eat my lunch and dinner I need to have 50% protein and 50% veg or salad. For breakfast I have two scrambled eggs with a glass of milk and a slice of tomato because eight weeks of scrambled eggs gets a bit hard to get down. I have that with a glass of milk and then the herbal tea that she gives me and then for lunch I have tuna and salad. I can have any meat except pork so I have fish and salad, meat and salad, chicken and salad, whatever - she didn't say quantities. I don't have a huge plate but I have about a handful of the protein and the same with the veg and then for dinner I have meat and veg. If we have spaghetti bolognaise I have the bolognaise but I don't have the spaghetti. I have vegetables or salad. No potatoes. I can have sweet potato and pumpkin so that's okay.

I noticed a difference in my energy levels. I feel much better. I've lost weight, about 6 or 7 kilos, so I feel better about myself and I have been doing exercise. I go running a couple of times a week just for 20 minutes and I feel more energetic about that and it seems much easier to do it and I don't have quite so many mood swings. I also don't have so many headaches.

Menstrual Changes

My periods are also getting shorter because they were around the 35 and above days and I would get to day 30 and I'd start spotting, then I'd stop, then I'd start spotting and then it just went on and on and then eventually I would get my period. Then that would go on for about seven days and so it was two weeks out of five I was bleeding. That has slowly shortened and not quite so much spotting so it is slowly getting better.

I'm feeling good but it is a struggle because every day there's temptation and it's that willpower to not have the particular food, so occasionally. On Mother's Day I went to my mother-in-law's for dinner and I had a piece of cake. But the sky didn't fall in and that's what my husband says. Well you didn't die did you? The TCM practitioner said that when I have a piece of cake, or whatever I eat that I think I shouldn't, to **watch my basal body temperature** *because I'll see the next day that it will either drop or go up. It actually does but it depends what I eat because at Easter I had two dark chocolate eggs, just the tiny ones, and the next day my temperature went up higher. The TCM practitioner said 'well that's good, that means, you can quite easily have dark chocolate if your temperature goes up in the second phase of your cycle because that's what we want so I do have a little bit of dark chocolate'.*

Diet Influences Basal Body Temperature, Fertility and General Well-being

Not having alcohol doesn't worry me. I have been having a couple of coffees a week because I love coffee and I meet with a group of friends I have a cup of coffee. I do let myself have that and that doesn't affect my temperature. It's probably not too bad.

My blood group doesn't allow me to have yoghurt, which I love, and I have had a few evenings where I've been really hungry and had a small serve of yoghurt which has affected my temperature. In the early part of the cycle, when it should stay low, yoghurt tends to put the temperature right up.

The TCM practitioner talks about getting your body back to wellness, that the food you eat does make a big difference to what you feel and how your body functions. I think the problem is that the way we live nowadays. There's so much temptation for food that isn't good for you and you get into that habit of eating that food. *But now we're all eating healthier because I'm eating healthier and I'm buying healthier, we don't have takeaway and we don't eat out because I think what's the point? I can just make something just as nice at home. We didn't eat a lot of takeaway before and we didn't eat out a lot before either but I used to have things in the house, cakes and biscuits. I still have those things occasionally for the kids. The kids have eaten less of it as I've got stricter with things. I say 'look that's not for every day, that's now and then'. So I'm trying to change their attitude as well that they can't eat that stuff whenever they want.*

One Step Forward, Two Steps Back

I got a bit frustrated with the second month because I was really strict and I had not eating anything bad and my temperature was very erratic. The TCM practitioner explained "that's the toxins in your body, you've still got three months you need for detoxing" so she said that's just my body's reaction to getting rid of the toxins.

My Experience with TCM Herbal Therapy

Taking the herbs doesn't worry me at all and my husband doesn't seem to be too worried about having the herbs. He thinks it's more of a natural kind of thing. He says he might even need to go and see the TCM practitioner. The first couple of weeks I thought it's a bit like taking muddy water with a mushroom kind of earthy taste. But now I actually quite like it. It's almost like having a black coffee. It's got that kind of taste to it. I actually don't mind taking it and I find that it does suppress my hunger a little bit when I have it. It also actually gives me a sense of power. If I actually start to ovulate myself, I do start to feel that I've got a bit more control over my body again.

If I did have another baby I would definitely go and see the TCM practitioner to get back to this again. If I became pregnant, I would continue to see the TCM practitioner during the pregnancy because from what she says that seems to be the most important part of it. The TCM practitioner has said to me that if I get pregnant I am not to do the glucose tolerance test. This is because of the way my pancreas and liver is, she said if I have that big hit of sugar, it may result like quite a few women who come back and have had miscarriages at that 32/31 weeks from that. She said don't do it, so I'm not sure how that will go but we'd have to just face that as it happens. It's my choice. It's not something that I'm obliged to do. I didn't have the test with the other children and my diet is so restricted that there's no way that I could have diabetes.

Part 4: Unexplained Infertility Explained

Unexplained infertility is accepted as a valid diagnosis in Western Medicine, with 20-25% of all couples dealing with infertility being affected. Couples have usually undergone routine fertility tests, including semen analysis and blood tests of women to check for fertility hormone levels. Additionally, some women might have been tested using pelvic ultrasound to check for ovarian cysts, or more invasive tests, such as laparoscopy (the abdominal cavity and pelvis are looked at through a small telescope inserted through the naval) or hysterosalpingo-contrast-sonography (HyCoSy) (a transvaginal ultrasound to investigate fallopian tube blockage). If no abnormalities are detected, couples often receive the diagnosis of 'unexplained infertility'.

This diagnosis of unexplained infertility can cause grief and distress by many couples. Some do not accept this as the last word spoken, and sometimes find their way to complementary and alternative health care practitioners. Naturopaths and Traditional Chinese Medicine (TCM) practitioners, in particular, offer a more holistic approach to fertility and general health. A holistic approach incorporates lifestyle factors, such as diet and general well-being. Manifestations of the menstrual cycle, including cycle length, BBT pattern, and menstruation itself can provide the key to underlying imbalances and causes for infertility, as the following stories by women with unexplained infertility illustrate.

Story 5: Temperature Charts

Bella explains how thorough observation of her basal body temperature pattern gave clues about underlying causes for her infertility. Bella was diagnosed with unexplained infertility after 3 years of investigations and trying. During that time she experienced a lot of grief.

Unexplained Infertility

We got married in March (2001), came of the Pill in April, expected to be pregnant by June and then a year later nothing happened. I was quite determined to try and find out what the problem was - I was 33 years old. I was increasingly anxious about the whole thing and disappointed.

We had two cycles of Intra-Uterine Insemination (IUI) which weren't successful. My husband's tests came back completely fine and I was completely fine - there was no impediment to conception as far as the doctors could find out but pregnancy still wasn't happening. I even had tests where they put dye through my tubes and made sure everything is fine, and it came back clear. It took ages – two or three years to conceive. Once we had been diagnosed with unexplained infertility - after three years of investigations and trying - we went private. They did a laparoscopy - that's using a camera to look into the uterus - and discovered some endometriosis, which they treated.

I experienced a lot of grief during that time, particularly because we had these IUI's and kept being told that, "Oh you're fine", and my age wasn't necessarily a factor and my husband is younger than I am, so everything was always thought to be positive and so every month I was hopeful, but then it just seemed to be not working. Nobody could say why. And at the same time, all of my friends were having babies and my brothers were having families, so there seemed to be lots of them about and however much I tried to be happy for other people, it's just hard.

Unexplained Explained
Regulating the Menstrual Cycle with TCM

Bella looked for alternative options to help her fall pregnant and found a TCM practitioner who explained that key to fertility is a regular menstrual cycle. This involves regular temperature pattern observable with the basal body temperature (BBT) chart, length of cycle, and also colour and flow of the menstrual blood itself.

I had TCM before (unrelated to fertility), and found acupuncture and herbal medicine completely effective, so I had a lot of faith in it. I'd read on the internet that Chinese Medicine was quite effective with infertility. So after a few months of trying to conceive and it not happening, I went to see this practitioner and he was fantastic. Because the whole process was very stressful, I found it incredibly important to have him to help, just to talk to. I was charting my temperature, using ovulation temperature charts, then over a period of months my temperature was all over the place. It didn't have a regular spike, it didn't follow a regular pattern and over those few months of treatment using acupuncture and herbal medicine, it settled into a much more regular classical kind of temperature, the spike just before you ovulate and then the dip and also my periods changed significantly.

My periods changed from the first two days being heavy and painful and dark blood and then very light for those three days following. After some months of treatment they became more steady in flow and a brighter red colour and far less painful, in fact the pain more or less went. And this was over a period of six or seven months, it changed like that.

Complementing of IVF Treatment with TCM

I kept seeing the Chinese Medicine practitioner throughout all the investigations and trying. He said that acupuncture could go alongside IVF, there are certain studies that show increases the potential of pregnancy. I went to see him on the day of implantation, he was quite critical about having to see him on that day at a certain time. I saw him all the way through and then when I got pregnant I saw him for morning sickness etc. Fortunately I got pregnant.

Any medically trained doctor would probably say IVF was what sorted it out, that's what got me pregnant but I'm sure that it wasn't. I feel that the acupuncture and the herbal medicine was significant in regulating my cycle and aiding conception and also helped psychologically, which is incredibly important, too.

Bella fell pregnant a second time. This time naturally.

My second wasn't an IVF baby. After our first daughter was born, we had some frozen embryos left over and we used those up and I didn't get pregnant. And then we moved and we went to a different IVF clinic and I had a round of IVF there and I got pregnant, but it was ectopic, and so I had a tube removed and I thought "oh well, that's it for us". But then a month or two later I just got pregnant naturally with my second. With one tube, at 38. After all this time.

Story 6: Low Temperature and Oligomenorrhea

Melanie's story highlights the importance of the 'ideal body temperature conducive for fertility and conception. Melanie always had long and irregular menstrual cycles ranging between 45 and 98 days on average. Prescribed treatment was the contraceptive pill. Melanie has been trying to fall pregnant for 3 years. She is 32 years old.

Unexplained Infertility

I went to a few doctors when I was trying to conceive with my ex-husband. They basically said it was unexplained. I had ultrasounds and there were no cysts, nothing on my ovaries, it can't be PCOS and it's not endometriosis. I was sent to a gynaecologist who also said it was unexplained and recommended that I take a fertility drug but I told him that I didn't want to do *that. From speaking to a lot of other women that have gone through unexplained infertility, they have been told to go on fertility drugs rather than be recommended alternative approaches or go further with their testing.*

I found it confusing, the doctors would tell you there was nothing wrong but there's obviously something wrong because your body is not doing what it's meant to be doing and how can that be unexplainable? How can I just be put on a drug even though I don't know what my body is doing? I found that doctors don't take a holistic approach. They're very quick to say 'It's unexplainable, let's just put you on drugs for it'. I had a classic example of a doctor late last year who I spoke to when I first started to query my irregular cycles. One of my cycles had gone for 40 days and I'd had my period for a week, it stopped for two days and I had spotting for another three or four days. So I asked him 'what could this possibly be?' He said 'it's probably just your cycle ending' and I said 'after I had my period for seven days and it stops for two days? All my cycles are around this.' He told me that if I was worried I should go back on the pill. I was so upset and angry because he hadn't even asked me if I was trying to conceive. I have been shopping around for a good doctor. The last one told me that my tests were fine and to come back in a few months if things are still not good.

Melanie is aware that her cycles need to be regulated to be able to conceive. She sought out a TCM practitioner inspired by a friend's success story. She is treated for oligomenorrhea and low basal body temperature (BBT) which might be due to an underactive thyroid.

Treating Oligomenorrhea and low BBT with TCM

I've been charting my cycles and that's what prompted me to go and see a TCM practitioner who does acupuncture and Chinese Medicine to try to help regulate my cycles so I can conceive. I had a friend tell me a story about her daughter's irregular cycles and her success with acupuncture. I then went online and did some research and decided I would like to try TCM rather than going down the IVF path because I don't like drugs. I rather try a natural alternative first. I like the holistic approach.

I have only been seeing the TCM practitioner for about five weeks. At the moment I'm finishing a detox of 10 days trying to clear out my system as well as having acupuncture and taking herbs and herbal tablets that she prescribes me. I am also treated for the symptoms of Polycystic Ovarian Syndrome because the practitioner thinks that I actually do have that condition. Even though the ultrasound does not show any cysts on my ovaries, I do have symptoms of the syndrome.

I'm not sure if my GP had tested my thyroid function but when I started seeing the TCM practitioner she got me to start charting my temperatures and it is around 36 degrees Celsius which indicates an underactive thyroid. So we're treating that with herbal tablets as well. I understand from some of the research I've done myself online that it's often difficult to tell if you have a thyroid condition especially if it doesn't come up on the normal tests, but further testing was never suggested to me by my GP, I was only ever told to come back in a couple of months hoping that it will just go away. It never did. It's very frustrating.

Story 7: High Temperature and Recurrent Miscarriages

The basal body temperature is important for fertility, whether the temperature is too low or too high impacts on the ability to conceive and carry a viable pregnancy. While Melanie's BBT was too low - around 36.0 degrees Celsius - as she described above, Rachel's BBT was too high causing her recurrent miscarriages. In fact, in TCM 'Cold or Heat in the body' are considered an imbalance which can be treated.

Rachel had lost four pregnancies early, when she decided to seek alternative therapies. Rachel recollects:

The TCM practitioner explained that I had a weakened qi, and my body was very hot and it needed to be cooled down. My body was not conducive to having a child because it was so hot and my body wasn't putting as much nutrients into my blood as it should. It makes sense to say that I'm too hot because I walk around in t-shirts when my partner and kids are in jumpers.

Story 8: Intestinal Candida

The following three stories highlight how diet and digestive health can influence fertility, conception and viable pregnancy.

Thalissa had been trying for a baby for 3 years and had experienced both a typical fertility clinic and a TCM clinic. TCM diagnostic suggested digestive issues and yeast (candida) overgrowth as possible cause for infertility.

Unexplained Infertility

After 8 months of trying, we were referred by the GP to a fertility specialist at an IVF practice. They carried out the testing, the semen analysis and I had the blood tests and the checks for ovulation, the HyCoSy test to check the tubes were open. We have had a lot of the basic tests done and they have all come back as normal, as far as they can tell. So we are officially unexplained. The specialist said "come back in six months time" and we haven't yet done that. The last appointment that we had there was about 2 years ago.

Then, we tried naturally for six months, and it was after about another six months since seeing the specialist I starting pursuing the line of preventative medicine and found a Traditional Chinese Medicine Clinic that specialises in infertility through the internet.

Holistic Approach to Infertility through TCM

In the TCM clinic I went through a whole health check. They aimed to identify a reason from a Chinese health perspective that might be causing fertility problems. They looked particularly at subjective issues and felt that my body was focussing on digestion rather than reproduction. Initially I was just having acupuncture once a week, after about three months I took the Chinese herbs in addition to the acupuncture. It was a ready-made powder to dilute with water.

Before I had the Chinese herbs they gave me probiotics and fish oil. This was to clear up some kind of yeast infection in the digestive tract. They recommended diet changes as well. In the beginning I was quite strict following their recommendations, which was no yeast, no wheat, no dairy, changing towards soy products and trying to balance the digestive system by getting in a variety of grains. Then after about three months I would start taking the Chinese herbs to boost my fertility.

In addition, I felt I was going to counselling but not in a counselling way. I talked about how I felt, and they were interested in how my week has been and how I was feeling and what my energy levels are like. There was much more opportunity just to talk with the TCM practitioners. They were quite interested in all the highs and lows of my week.

In contrast to western fertility clinics, the menstrual cycle pattern is integrated in the holistic approach.

At my first appointment with the western fertility specialist, I had taken in some of my charts and thinking that he might be interested in looking at ovulation patterns or else and he just went "oh yes, very nice". Not quite as blunt I guess but it was more about "ok, these are the tests that I can do, which ones are we going to give you".

On the other hand the TCM practitioner said "bring in all the charts that you have done. Let's have a look, if we need to extend the luteal phase, or if ovulation is around the right time..."

Story 9: Candida and Temperature

33-year old Susi has been trying to get pregnant for about five years and was diagnosed with unexplained infertility. Her disbelieve in 'unexplained infertility' and interest in holistic approaches has encouraged her to lose weight. Furthermore, she found a TCM practitioner who encouraged her to follow an anti-candida diet.

Unexplained Infertility

When I was having trouble having a baby, I saw my doctor and I said to her, "Can I see somebody?" and she sent me to one of the fertility specialists and he did all the exploratory stuff, the camera in there and having a look around (laparoscopy) and he said I had a beautiful uterus. There's no endometriosis, there's no reason why. You're in the unexplained category and here's the number for the IVF clinic.

I thought okay, I don't know if that's right because normally there's a reason why. ***I don't believe in unexplained****, there's got to be some reason and then I thought to myself, if I can't get pregnant normally then I don't think IVF would help because obviously whatever's wrong might stop that from working as well and I didn't see the point in doing that.*

I found it odd when the specialist said it to me "Have you tried any of those ovulation kits?" and I said, "Yeah I tried it once but there was no success". "Have you been taking your temperature?" and I said, "Yeah I've been doing that" and I actually showed him and the specialist goes, "Well I don't believe in that sort of thing".

Unexplained Explained

Susi explains what motivated her to lose weight and how she achieved that. She also outlines how observation of her low BBT indicates candida overgrowth in the digestive system.

I felt that the specialist had washed his hands off me. He said "I've done all I can do in that I've looked inside you, and my husband's sperm are fine, that's all I can do." Not once did the specialist say, "It could be something that you're eating" because at that stage I was a little bit heavier as well. When I first went to see him and he said unexplained I thought, "No, that's not good enough, it's got to be something" and I lost 15 kilos.

At that time there were some stories on TV about naturopaths. I read Ruth Sharkey's books saying weight could be a factor too. I thought, "Fair enough, I'm not going to be overweight anymore".

I cut out, I needed to understand some of the foods that I was eating. My serving sizes were too big and my eating times were all over the place because I did shift work back then as well. And that cook book came out, that was my saviour. I followed that to the letter, day one to day 12 and I lost so much weight just in that first few months and I started understanding food. But I'm not there yet. I'm not where I want to be. I still want maybe another five or six kilos and I'm just working on that and the TCM practitioner is helping me as well which is good. "Take potatoes off." "Oh no but I love potatoes" "Don't eat it so much." I'm not eating it so much now. This is a treat, this is the size.

In addition, my Mum was seeing a TCM practitioner just to feel better, lose a bit of weight. Maybe, I thought, the TCM practitioner might be able to help with fertility.

On contrast to the fertility specialist, the TCM practitioner was interested in my charts. She was very positive. She checked my pulse on my wrists and was interested in what I ate and she goes, "I know your problem. I'm going to be able to get you pregnant really soon" and she seemed really positive. She seemed to think that I had a yeast infection like thrush but inside (candida overgrowth) that no-one picked up. So she's taken me off wheat. I didn't know there was so much wheat in the foods you eat. I'm learning a lot about that. I started doing that about two months ago. I'm in a 5 week follow-up now with her because she wants to see me after the next period starts. So I started seeing her then and she was saying, "Go off wheat and fix your diet up and lose a bit of weight". That sounds good. I'm all for weight loss. I started the herbal teas the last time that I saw her because the first time she said, "I just want you off wheat to see if we can get these toxins out of you" and to track my temperature so I went and bought a thermometer and I've tracked that and she showed me the BBT charts – the charts recording your temperature and any changes you see in your cervix and your mucus discharge.

My TCM practitioner picked up where I'm ovulating and so she showed that to me at the last appointment and she goes, "You're definitely ovulating around here". She gave me herbs, tea, there's one for the first part of the cycle and one for the second part.

She said to me, "Day 15 is when you start this next one". She seemed to think that I'm ovulating okay but my temperatures are very low. She said the seed (eggs) is not great and the soil (body environment) is not great so she's given me some herbs to work on that because my temperatures are low, 35.8s and 35.9s, when they should have been 36.2, around there. She said that it was too low.

I am feeling generally better in myself since I've started seeing the TCM practitioner. I always felt really bloated and really heavy and tired. But after sticking to the anti-candida diet, my energy levels got up a little bit. I felt a bit happier about things and I don't feel that heaviness anymore in the stomach. And I definitely feel more hopeful.

Story 10: Inflammation and Food Intolerance

Diana has been trying for a baby for more than five years, since she got married at 37. She thought to fall pregnant straight away but it didn't happen. Her periods came every 28 to 35 days but were very light. She has sought help at an IVF clinic, and had five cycles of IVF, two in a year. While she fell pregnant, she miscarried at 6 to 9 weeks of gestation when using IVF. She recollects her experience being told that her inability to carry a viable pregnancy was unexplained.

I had every test known to man. Most times the specialists couldn't find what was wrong but then they did a biopsy of my uterus and they said that was all inflamed, and he gave me some antibiotics, and actually fixed it and said "we'll try another cycle", but it still didn't work. The specialist said, "sometimes these miscarriages are just unexplained" and I went,

"No, do not say that". He said, "I think you should consider adoption" or something like that. I said, "There's obviously something wrong there that's making my uterus inflamed - just because you can't find it, there has got to be more tests".

And obviously if something is wrong, it's affecting my health elsewhere, not just trying to get pregnant. I've been checked for literally every disease twice a year for the last five years so we knew it was none of those. They just don't know. The specialist said: "I can't help you." We ended up with an operation to look inside (laparoscopy). There was a lot of scarring in my uterus.

Meanwhile Diana has sought advice from a TCM practitioner who was recommended to her by a friend. The TCM practitioner suspects underlying gluten intolerance causing Diana's problems. In addition, Diana has continued to visit her naturopath.

The TCM practitioner suggested gluten intolerance, which could cause inflammation. She's got me on cleansing teas to detox my body. I'm on a gluten-free diet and I eat more meat, more vegetables - I wasn't a big meat eater. Now I feel better, I feel healthier. I've lost a bit of weight.

A naturopath, I've seen earlier, had also suggested cleansing my body, and advised to reduce stress. My job is indeed stressful. I heard that the stress creates a hormone (cortisol) that can affect your uterus.

The TCM practitioner has been very positive. She said 'the body is an amazing thing and the uterus lining, it changes all the time, it will repair itself with the right treatment." She said not to worry. She explained that, for example, Crohn's Disease primarily affects the bowels, however if it can affect the bowels, it can affect any part of the body. The uterus is a body part. Women shed the endometrial lining, and then it is renewed.

I also saw my naturopath a month ago. I had some more tests done and she said my oestrogen level was lower than normal, and gave me something to help boost the oestrogen level. When I went to the TCM practitioner yesterday, and showed her my BBT charts, she said, "your oestrogen is too low", because of temperature pattern in my chart. The naturopath and the TCM practitioners said the same thing without seeing the other's results.

Acknowledgments

I am indebted to my colleague and friend Dr Ann Alfred, who conducted the interviews with the women and provided a sounding board during this project. We are grateful to all the women who participated and to the TCM practitioner Jenny Chou who helped with the recruitment of several women for this project.

References

[1] ACCESS. Australia's National Infertility Network. Available from: http://www.access.org.au.

[2] RESOLVE. The National Infertility Association, Virginia, USA. Available from: http://www.resolve.org.

[3] Wang YA, Macaldowie A, Hayward I, Chambers GM, Sullivan EA. Assisted reproductive technology in Australia and New Zealand 2009. *Assisted reproduction technology series no 15 Cat no PER 51*. Canberra: Australian Institute of Health and Welfare, 2011.

[4] van Gool K, Savage E, Johar M, Knox S, Jones G, Viney R. Australian Government Department of Health and Ageing. Extended Medicare Safety Net benefit caps for assisted reproductive technology items. MBS Online 2011. Available from: http://www.health.gov.au/internet/ mbsonline/publishing.nsf/Content/Factsheet-EMSN-1_Jan_2011.

[5] IVFAustralia. Our current costs. 2011. Available from: http://www.ivf. com.au/ivf-treatment-costs/our-current-costs.aspx

[6] Greil AL. Infertility and psychological distress: a critical review of the literature. *Soc Sci Med*. 1997; 45: 1679-704.

[7] Imeson M, McMurray A. Couples' experiences of infertility: a phenomenological study. *J Adv Nurs*. 1996; 24: 1014-22.

[8] Redshaw M, Hockley C, Davidson LL. A qualitative study of the experience of treatment for infertility among women who successfully became pregnant. *Hum Reprod*. 2007; 22: 295-304.

[9] McCarthy MP. Women's lived experience of infertility after unsuccessful medical intervention. *J Midwifery Womens Health*. 2008; 53: 319-24.

[10] Malik SH, Coulson NS. Computer-mediated infertility support groups: an exploratory study of online experiences. *Patient Educ Couns*. 2008; 73: 105-13.

[11] Alfred A, Ried K. Traditional Chinese Medicine - Women's experiences in the treatment of infertility. *Aust Fam Physician*. 2011; 40: 718-22.

[12] Albertson K. The use of Traditional Chinese Medicine for treating female infertility. Birmingham, Alabama: Clayton College of Natural Health, 2006.

[13] Charles J, Pan Y, Britt H. Management of infertility in Australian general practice. *Aust Fam Physician*. 2005; 34: 104-5.

[14] Noll AA, Wilms S. *Chinese Medicine in Fertility Disorders*. Stuttgart: Thieme, 2010.

[15] Maciocia G. *Obsterics and Gynecology in Chinese Medicine*. London: Churchill Livingston, 1998.

[16] Lyttleton J. *Treatment of Infertility with Chinese Medicine*. London: Churchill Livingston, 2004.

[17] Lewis R. *The infertility cure: The ancient Chinese wellness program for getting pregnant and having healthy babies*. New York: Little, Brown and Company, 2004.

[18] Kaptchuk T. *Chinese Medicine: the web that has no weaver*. Essex: Anchor Brendon Ltd, 1983.

[19] Wood V. Infertility and the use of basal body temperature in diagnosis and treatment. *Journal of Chinese Medicine*. 1999; 61: 33-41.

[20] Ried K, Stuart K. Efficacy of Traditional Chinese Herbal Medicine in the management of female infertility: A systematic review. *Complement Ther Med*. 2011; 19: 319-31.

[21] Higgins JPT, Green S, (editors). Cochrane Handbook for Systematic Reviews of Interventions Version 5.0.2. The Cochrane Collaboration 2009. Available from: www.cochrane-handbook.org.

[22] Victorian Assisted Reproductive Treatment Authority. Annual Report 2010. Melbourne, VIC.

[23] Chavarro JE, Rich-Edwards JW, Rosner BA, Willett WC. Diet and lifestyle in the prevention of ovulatory disorder infertility. *Obstet Gynecol*. 2007; 110: 1050-8.

[24] Heese I. The 'egg factor': Using Chinese herbal medicine to improve fertility in a 45-year old women. *J Chin Med*. 2006; 82: 36-41.

[25] See CJ, McCulloch M, Smikle C, Gao J. Chinese herbal medicine and clomiphene citrate for anovulation: a meta-analysis of randomized controlled trials. *J Altern Complement Med*. 2011; 17: 397-405.

[26] Nader S. Infertility and pregnancy in women with polycystic ovary syndrome. *Minerva Endocrinol*. 2010; 35: 211-25.

[27] de Ziegler D, Borghese B, Chapron C. Endometriosis and infertility: pathophysiology and management. *Lancet*. 2010; 376: 730-8.

[28] Zhang X. Traditional Chinese Medicine and Laparoscopic surgery for the management of Endometriosis. *Asia Pacific Endometriosis Alliance Newsletter*. 2006: 1-4.

[29] Chambers GM, Ho MT, Sullivan EA. Assisted reproductive technology treatment costs of a live birth: an age-stratified cost-outcome study of treatment in Australia. *Med J Aust*. 2006; 184: 155-8.

[30] AACMA. Australasian Acupuncture and Chinese Medicine Association. Available from: http://www.acupuncture.org.au.

[31] *Chinese Medicine Registration Board of Victoria*. Available from: www.cmrb.vic.gov.au.

In: Infertility
Editors: R. Nascimento and H. V. Boas

ISBN: 978-1-62257-909-9

Chapter 2

Adverse Outcomes of Assisted Reproduction Techniques

Bruno Ramalho de Carvalho, Taciana Fontes Rolindo, David Barreira Gomes Sobrinho, Hitomi Miura Nakagava, Adelino Amaral Silva, Antônio César Paes Barbosa, Marcel Eiji Miura Nakagava and Marco Akio Miura Nakagava
GENESIS – Center for Assistance in Human Reproduction,
Brasília, DF, Brazil

Abstract

From the first birth of a child conceived by in vitro fertilization (IVF), much has been developed in assisted reproduction techniques (ART). However, the evolution of knowledge and therapeutic options, and progressively better results, were not followed by a proper control of risks and complications, which are still considerably frequent. The aim of this chapter is to deeply discuss undesirable outcomes such as ovarian hyperstimulation syndrome, ectopic and multiple pregnancies, and the higher rates of miscarriage among patients submitted to ART. In addition, birth defects, epigenetic inheritance and perinatal outcomes will be discussed, with the aim to offer clinicians an updated reference for daily practice.

Introduction

Assisted reproduction techniques (ART) started a new era in reproductive medicine, when, more than 30 years ago, resulted in the first *in vitro* conceived child in England. Since then, technological development has promoted increased success rates. It is estimated that approximately 5 million ART-conceived babies were born in the world until today (ESHRE, 2012).

According to the European Society of Human Reproduction and Embriology (ESHRE), around 1.5 million ART cycles are performed worldwide each year, resulting in approximately 350.000 births. In Nordic countries and Belgium, ART result in up to 3.0% of all births. Although results statistics are similar between the most performed commonly used techniques, conventional *in vitro* fertilization (IVF) now accounts now for almost one-third and intracytoplasmic sperm injection (ICSI) contributes with two-thirds of all cycles (ESHRE, 2012).

Even though much has been developed in ART, there are still many uncertainties to be clarified. Studies to investigate the mechanisms involved in embryo implantation, for example, may offer valuable contribution to the achievement of pregnancy by transferring a single embryo, thus reducing the chances of multiple pregnancy and its complications. Similarly, studies of large populations conceived by IVF/ICSI will be increasingly feasible, contributing not only with more reliable evaluation of the psychomotor development of those children, but offering answers to questions concerning the incidence of defects in imprinting or epigenetic changes.

Once the evolution of knowledge and therapeutic options, and progressively better results of ART were not followed by a proper control of risks and complications, the aim of this chapter is to deeply discuss undesirable outcomes, such as ovarian hyperstimulation syndrome (OHSS), ectopic and multiple pregnancies, and the higher rates of miscarriage among patients submitted to ART. Also, birth defects, epigenetic inheritance and perinatal outcomes will be discussed, offering clinicians an updated rationale for daily practice.

Ovarian Hyperstimulation Syndrome

Ovarian hyperstimulation syndrome (OHSS) is one of the most worrisome complications of ART. It is expected that OHSS occurs in 0.5 to 5% of all ovarian stimulation cycles and in up to 10% of IVF cycles (D'Angelo and Amso, 2007). However, as this disorder and its complications are not always predictable, prevention of severe cases is a concern of ART services.

The pathophysiology of OHSS is marked by increased capillary permeability, leading to the accumulation of protein and fluids outside the vascular compartment; despite the lack of knowledge on its exact mechanisms, it is supposed that mediation by vasoactive cytokines secreted by the luteal body in response to human chorionic gonadotropin (hCG) stimulation has a major participation (Chen et al., 2010). Proinflammatory cytokynes and vascular endothelial growth factor (VEGF) have been correlated with the development of OHSS and its severity.

Diagnosis

Ascites with abdominal and pelvic pain or discomfort are the most common symptoms of OHSS, and the accumulation of hyperproteic fluid in the peritoneal cavity leads to abdominal distention and increased intra-abdominal pressure (abdominal compartment syndrome), with deleterious consequences on respiratory, cardiovascular, renal, gastrointestinal and hepatic functions. Also, hypotension, tachycardia, hemoconcentration and hypercoagulability are expected as results of a depletion in the intravascular volume. In severe cases, arterial and venous thrombosis, hepatorenal failure, hydroelectrolyte imbalances, pleural and/or pericardial effusion, acute respiratory distress syndrome and hemorrhage from ovarian rupture may occur (The Practice Committee of the American Society for Reproductive Medicine, 2008a; Humaidan et al., 2010). Some investigational tests are important to diagnose and evaluate the imbalance grade with OHSS severity: serum electrolytes, creatinine and proteins; hemogram; coagulogram; liver function; 24 hours diuresis; pelvic, abdominal and thoracic sonography.

In spite of being a dynamic disease, OHSS has been classified by clinical and laboratorial manifestations to determine its severity and evolution. OHSS may be firstly distinguished by time of onset. Early OHSS is caused by exogenous hCG administered for follicular final maturation and it is usually diagnosed from 3 to 7 days after trigger; once pregnancy does not occur, it usually disappears with menses. OHSS with onset 12 or more days after the ovulatory injection of hCG is classified as late and is developed as a consequence of the endogenous hCG secretion in an ongoing early pregnancy (Mathur et al., 2000); it is given to evolve into a severe syndrome and may last around 12 weeks.

Based on the laboratory and clinical disturbances OHSS may also be classified into three categories: mild, moderate or severe. According to the American Society for Reproductive Medicine (ASRM), severe OHSS is defined by the presence of abdominal pain plus at least one of the following signs or symptoms: rapid weight gain, respiratory distress, oliguria, hemodynamic instability (orthostatic hypotension, tachycardia), tense ascites, hemoconcentration (hematocrit > 45%), leukocytosis (white blood cell count > 15,000), elevated liver enzymes, serum creatinine > 1.2 mg/dL, hyponatremia (Na < 135 mEq/L) and hyperkalemia (K > 5.0 mEq/L) (The Practice Committee of the American Society for Reproductive Medicine, 2008a).

Treatment and Prevention

Mild and most of the moderate cases presenting no jeopardized biochemical or hematologic parameters can be assisted in an outpatient system with conservative management. Hospitalization and intensive care should be considered when at least one of the following events arise: severe abdominal pain or peritoneal signs, intractable nausea and vomiting that prevents adequate ingestion of food and fluids, severe oliguria or anuria, tense ascites, dyspnea or tachypnea, hypotension (relative to baseline), dizziness or syncope, severe electrolyte hyponatremia or hyperkalemia), hemoconcentration, abnormal liver function tests (The Practice Committee of the American Society for Reproductive Medicine, 2008a; Budev et al., 2005).

OHSS prevention is one of the cornerstones in ART. The primary prevention strategy is based on: (1) evaluation of patients' ovarian reserve; (2) identification of risk factors; and (3) adequacy of stimulation protocol. Antimüllerian hormone dosage (AMH) and sonographic antral follicle count (AFC) are the ovarian reserve tests of choice; AMH cut-off value of 3.36 ng/mL and AFC cut off level of > 14 follicles predicted OHSS occurrence with sensitivity of 90.5% and 82%, respectively (Lee et al., 2008). Age < 35 years, low body mass index, polycystic ovary syndrome, history of atopy or allergies, and previous episode of OHSS are also recognized as pre-treatment identifiable risk factors (Delvigne and Rozenberg, 2002; Delvigne, 2009). Finally, the protocol of choice for those potential high-responders must be the GnRH antagonist protocol with the lower possible dose of gonadotropins for ovarian stimulation, which has been shown to significantly minimize the incidence and severity of OHSS (Al-Inany et al., 2011).

Some aspects should help clinicians to apply secondary prevention strategies during controlled ovarian hyperstimulation: estradiol levels ≥ 5000 pg/mL; total follicular count ≥ 20 follicles; or 13 or more follicles with diameter ≥ 11mm (Papanikolaou et al., 2006). Reduction of the dose of gonadotropins or administration of the triggering bolus of hCG earlier may decrease the risk of OHSS by inducing the regression of small and medium sized follicles (Papanikolaou et al., 2011). The coasting strategy may also be adopted in cases of OHSS risk, allowing fresh embryo transfer with acceptable outcomes. The optimum time to start coasting is when the leading follicle diameter reaches 16 mm. After withdrawing gonadotropins, it is expected that functioning granulosa cell cohort diminishes, intermediary follicles become atretic and E2 serum levels fall. hCG may then be administered when E2 level drops below 3000 pg/ml. However, it is important to remember that premature coasting may lead to follicular arrest and that a decrease in pregnancy rates is noted when gonadotropin-free period lasts more than three days (Aboulghar, 2012).

Once there is no clear evidence that earlier or low-dose hCG would completely reduce OHSS, triggering ovulation by the administration of a GnRH agonist (GnRHa) (0.2 mg Triptorelin or 0.5 mg Buserelin or 1 mg Leuprolide) is an innovative and effective way applicable in the antagonist protocol to reduce its occurrence (Kol et al., 2000; Kol et al., 2012). Triggering ovulation with GnRHa and performing a complete embryo freeze should eliminate the chances of OHSS and offer high ongoing pregnancy rates in subsequent frozen-thawed transfer cycles (Kol et al., 2012).

Other drugs have been used to prevent or reduce consequences of OHSS, but conflicting findings do not allow consensual positions. In PCOS patients, metformin seems to reduce the risk of OHSS by modulating ovarian response to gonadotropins (Palomba et al., 2011) and it is also suggested that those patients would have higher live birth rates in subsequent frozen embryo transfer cycles (Brewer et al., 2010).

Based on the knowledge that dopamine agonists inhibits phosphorylation of the VEGF receptor-2 (Gomez et al., 2006), prophylactic low dose of cabergoline have shown a decrease in the incidence and severity of OHSS (Tehraninejad et al., 2012), but nine patients must be treated with the drug to prevent one case of OHSS (Youssef et al., 2010). In a recent review, Soares (2012) highlighted that a previous history of OHSS may indicate dopamine agonist use even with less evident signs of a strong ovarian response. The author recommended that oral daily dose of 0.5 mg cabergoline must be initiated ideally few hours before hCG administration and be maintained for 8 days. Rectal bromocriptine at a daily dose of 2.5 mg for 16 days is also a supported protocol (Soares, 2012).

Finally, as a plasma-binding protein, albumin may diminish vasoactive agents action and as an osmotic agent, it could help to avoid fluid shift from vessels and attenuate the effects of hypovolemia, hemoconcentration and ascites (Humaidan et al., 2010; Youssef et al., 2012). Nausea, vomiting, febrile or allergic reaction, anaphylactic shock and risk of virus and prion transmission are some of the undesirable side effects. According to Aboulghar et al. (2002), the number needed to treat to save one severe case of OHSS is eighteen (Aboulghar et al.,

2002) and Youssef et al. (2012) found a borderline statistically significant reduction in the incidence of severe OHSS in women treated with human albumin (Youssef et al., 2012).

Ectopic Pregnancy

Instinctively, it should be pertinent to believe that the occurrence of ectopic pregnancy (EP) is unlikely as embryos are transferred into the uterine cavity, however this was firstly described by Steptoe and Edwards in 1976 as a complication of the second attempt to obtain a pregnancy by IVF (Steptoe and Edwards, 1976). A Japanese group observed endometrial contractile movements progressing from internal os to the uterine fundus, secondary to high levels of estradiol (Milki and Jun, 2003). Such contractions should be responsible for moving transferred embryos into the fallopian tube (Jun and Milki, 2007). Augmented risk for EP is also expected with transcervical puncture (Lesny et al., 1999) or even excessive genital manipulation. Therefore, it is pertinent to consider that difficult transfers with cervical traction with Pozzi forceps or by the use of dilators may predispose to ectopic pregnancy. Initial studies indicated an incidence of 1 to 13% for EP after ART (The Practice Committee of the American Society for Reproductive Medicine, 2008b). Also, heterotopic pregnancies, characterized by the combination of an intrauterine pregnancy and one extrauterine, is supposed to be 70 times more common in women who have IVF for tubal factor.

The problem seems to be less frequent these days, corresponding to 1.8% for IVF and GIFT, and 4.3% for ZIFT cycles (Society for Assisted Reproductive Technology and the American Society for Reproductive Medicine, 2007). Despite performing ultrasound visualization does not seem to reduce EP rates (Fernandez and Gervaise, 2004), diminished frequency is probably due to improvements in the techniques of embryo transfer, and treatment of tubal disease, such as hydrosalpinx. Fortunately, early diagnosis is usually what makes the conservative treatment reliable.

Diagnosis

Pain and abnormal bleeding in patients submitted to ART with a positive test may be symptoms/signs of EP and should be precociously evaluated, once a delay in diagnosis may predispose to undesired complications of severe hemorrhage (Fernandes et al., 2004). Differential diagnosis must be held with miscarriage, rupture of hemorrhagic corpus luteum, salpingitis, anexial torsion, degenerative leiomyoma, endometriosis, appendicitis, abnormal uterine bleeding due to several conditions.

Human Chorionic Gonadotropin

Human chorionic gonadotropin (β-hCG) levels may be interpreted distinctly for pregnancies after ART compared to spontaneous ones, once it is known that ART themselves or the cause of infertility or both may affect the β-hCG concentration course (Fernandez and Gervaise, 2004).

Precocious sub-optimal levels of ß-hCG may be suggestive of EP. According to the study of Bjercke et al., β-hCG level < 55 mIU/mL on day 12 after embryo transfer was significantly associated with biochemical and extra-uterine pregnancies or first trimester abortions without permitting the differential diagnosis among them(Bjercke et al., 1999). An early post embryo transfer β-hCG level between 50 and 150 mIU/mL is supposed to yield a positive predictive value for pregnancy of 90% (Fernandez and Gervaise, 2004) and with levels around 200 mIU/mL at day 12 after embryo transfer, miscarriages are rarely expected and EP may be considered practically non-existent (Poikkeus et al., 2002).

Finally, a normal intrauterine pregnancy is expected to be identifiable by transvaginal ultrasound (TVUS) with β-hCG levels above the discriminatory zone of 1,500 to 2,500 mIU/mL. In the absence of an intrauterine gestational sac when the β-hCG serum concentration is above those values, an abnormal pregnancy may be present (The Practice Committee of the American Society for Reproductive Medicine, 2008c).

Transvaginal Ultrasound

Despite being an essential investigative method in the diagnosis of EP, TVUS is an operator-dependent exam, requiring considerable expertise in interpreting findings. Particularly after ART, hyperstimulated ovaries, ascites, endometriomas, hydrosalpinx or other common findings in infertile women make it difficult to identify the precise diagnosis. Then, systematic and attentive adnexal examination is required, even if one or more conceptus is topically developing, since 1–3% of IVF pregnancies are heterotopic. Nonetheless the low sensitivity, TVUS is expected to identify two-thirds of EP prior to rupture (Fernandez and Gervaise, 2004).

Treatment

Appropriate physical exam, ultrasound evaluation and complementary tests (complete blood count, liver enzymes, urea and creatinine, and blood typing) may help physicians to determine medical or surgical treatment, or expectant management of EP. Because of the risk of interstitial pneumonitis, women presenting prior pulmonary disease are also recommended to have a chest x-ray (The Practice Committee of the American Society for Reproductive Medicine, 2008c).

Medical Treatment

Methotrexate (MTX) administration should be indicated as the first therapeutic option. The main criteria for MTX administration are hemodynamic stability, β-hCG < 5,000 mUI/mL, adnexal mass < 3.5 to 4.0 cm, no alive embryo, absence of severe or persistent abdominal pain, normal liver and kidney functions, commitment to follow-up until the ectopic pregnancy has resolved and desire for future pregnancy. However, factors like TVUS detection of fetal cardiac activity, initial β-hCG > 5,000 mIU/mL, declining β-hCG titers in 24 to 48 hours (before treatment), refusal to receive blood transfusions with a written consent form signed, and the impossibility of follow-up should be considered for declining medical therapy. The absolute contraindications for MTX use are: intra-uterine pregnancy; immunodeficiency; moderate to severe anemia, leukopenia (white blood cells < 2000 cells/mm^3) or thrombocytopenia (platelets < 100,000); prior sensitivity to MTX; current pulmonary disease, peptic ulcer, hepatic and renal dysfunction; and breastfeeding (Elito Junior et al., 2008; The Practice Committee of the American Society for Reproductive Medicine, 2008c).

A single intramuscular MTX dose of 50 mg/m^2 is an effective and practical protocol, with fewer side effects. The follow-up must be taken through determining β-hCG serum titers on days 0, 4 and 7 from MTX administration, and the evident reduction 15% between days 4 and 7 must be considered as marker of good prognosis; β-hCG serum titers should be accompanied weekly until they reach pre-gravidic level. When the reduction is less than 15% on the seventh day after the use of MTX, a new dose of MTX must be provided. Protocol with multiple doses (1 mg/kg intramuscular, days 0, 2, 4, and 6, alternated with folinic acid 0.1 mg/kg, days 1, 3, 5, 7) should be preferred for cases with EP atypical localization (interstitial, cervical, caesarean section scar and ovarian pregnancies) or those with values of β-hCG > 5,000 mUI/mL and no alive embryo. Also, MTX may be applied as local treatment with an injection guided by TVUS in cases of alive embryos, but with an atypical localization (Elito Junior et al., 2008; The Practice Committee of the American Society for Reproductive Medicine, 2008c).

According to the meta-analysis of Mol et al., the results of two trials comparing a single MTX dose *versus* a fixed multiple dose protocol, showed no significant difference in EP treatment success (RR 0.99, 95% CI 0.89-1.10) (Klauser et al., 2005; Alleyassin et al., 2006), which means that there are insufficient data for a preferred protocol regarding treatment success, side effects or patients' health-related quality of life (Mol et al., 2008).

Surgical Treatment

Laparoscopic surgery is acceptable as the ideal route and most effective treatment in women with tubal EP (Mol et al., 2008; Elito Junior et al., 2008). Concerning surgical morbidity and mainly the reproductive future, controversies are raised between salpingectomy and salpingostomy. According to Elito Junior et al., salpingectomy should be the preferred approach for patients who have the desired number of children, while salpingostomy should be indicated to patients who are willing to conceive in the future (Elito Junior et al., 2008).

Expectant Management

According to Mol et al., no conclusions can be drawn from the single trial on expectant management (Mol et al., 2008). Criteria for expectant management are: no alive embryo, stable aspect in TVUS, and β-hCG decline in the 24 to 48 hours without treatment, when the initial levels are < 1.500 mIU/mL (Elito Junior et al., 2008).

Multiple Pregnancy

Undoubtedly, multiple pregnancies are concerning adverse results, which arise in the setting of ART and are directly related with the number of embryos transferred per cycle; the incidence varies from 23% in Europe (Andersen et al., 2008) to 32% in the United States (Wright et al., 2005). According to *Red Latinoamericana de Reproducción Asistida*, it is estimated that double pregnancies occur in up to 23% of cycles with two to four embryos transferred and in 5% of those with three to four embryos transferred (Zegers-Hochschild et al., 2008).

In the classic study of Schieve et al., the maximum IVF live birth rates among women < 35 years of age were achieved when two embryos were transferred to the uterus, but older patients needed more than 2 embryos to increase live birth rates. According to those authors, multiple-birth rate among women aged 30 to 34 years increased from 19.7% to 29.4% when 2 and 3 embryos were transferred, respectively; that rate raised from 11.6% to 29.4% among women aged 35 to 39 years, however, it was less than 25% for women aged 40 to 44 years, even if 5 embryos were transferred (Schieve et al., 1999).

Risks of multiple births from IVF vary by number of embryos transferred and maternal age. The birth of singletons or, at most, twins per treatment cycle is, undoubtedly, the optimal and rationale goal of ART, and can be easily accomplished by transferring one or two embryos per cycle. Since there is a negative interference of aging on IVF success rates (Abreu et al., 2006; Luna et al., 2007; Carvalho et al., 2010; Carvalho et al. 2012), it is acceptable to distinguish limits for numbers of embryos to be transfered according to age groups.

In Brazil, it is currently recommended to transfer a maximum of two embryos to women aged < 36 years, three embryos to women aged 36-39 years and four embryos to those aged > 39 years, with no possibility of increasing numbers, even in cases of repeated unsuccessful IVF cycles. The limits recommended for oocytes transferred in gamete intrafallopian transfer cycles is the same of those adopted for embryos (BRASIL/CFM, 2010).

An elective single embryo transfer (eSET) is a modern and widely accepted strategy for reducing multiple pregnancies, especially in blastocyst stage (Mullin et al., 2012) and mainly in countries where governments cover ART expenses. Moreover, advances in cryopreservation allow clinics to preserve the remaining embryos and warrant secure future transfers. A recent example was demonstrated in Finland, where eSET with cryopreservation was associated to a twofold reduction in multiple births, demonstrating to be more effective and less expensive than double embryo transfer (Veleva et al., 2009). Unfortunately, such a strategy is relatively uncommon in Brazil and the United States, where patients normally endure costs, discouraging the good prognostic couples and doctors from choosing it as a therapeutic plan.

Adverse perinatal outcomes such as low birth weight (LBW), preterm delivery (PTD) and fetal death are strongly attributable to multiple gestations. According to Chung et al. (2006), twin gestations were associated with a concerning 12-fold increased risk of LBW and/or PTD compared to singletons, and nearly all triplet pregnancies evolved with such complications (Chung et al., 2006), supporting the findings of other reports (Zegers-Hochschild et al., 2008; Nelson and Lawlor, 2011).

A higher risk of adverse obstetric outcomes in IVF singletons arises in the setting of spontaneous reductions from twin to singleton pregnancies (Pinborg et al., 2005).

Perinatal Outcomes

The association between ART and risk of undesirable perinatal outcomes such as LBW, PTD and fetal death is supported by a great body of evidence in literature; while those events are in part attributable to multiple pregnancies (Chung et al., 2006; Zegers-Hochschild et al., 2008; Nelson and Lawlor, 2011), an increased risk is also expected for singleton pregnancies.

In the study by Chung et al., type of gonadotropins used for ovulation induction or cumulative doses, treatment duration, serum estradiol (E2) peak, total number of dominant follicles, serum LH concentration, number of embryos transferred were not associated with LBW or PTD. Also, those authors did not find negative interference of the quality of embryos, the use of ICSI or assisted hatching or the etiology of infertility on infant outcomes. OHSS was associated with a fourfold increased risk for such adverse outcomes. Endometrial thickness seemed to be a protective factor for adverse perinatal outcomes, presenting with a more than twofold-increased risk in patients with endometrial measurements $\leq$ 10 mm when compared to those with more than 12 mm (Chung et al., 2006).

According with Klemetti et al., stillbirths are significantly more frequent among IVF-conceived children (7.2 cases per 1000 births), who also presented worse indicators of perinatal health; curiously, perinatal health of IVF multiples was comparable to that of naturally conceived multiples (Klemetti et al., 2006). Finally, in the recent study of Davies et al., women submitted to ART were more likely to have a stillbirth; also, ART was associated to higher incidences of cesarean section, preterm and extreme preterm births (Davies et al., 2012).

Children Conceived by ART

Over the past two decades, several studies have been published on the health and development of children conceived by ART, driven by concerns or ambiguous results on their normal evolution, particularly those in which IVF involved ICSI. However, current knowledge support physicians to advise future parents that ART-conceived singletons will probably develop in a very similar way of children born after spontaneous conception.

Birth Defects

Since the association between ART and birth defects was firstly raised, controversies have been frequently presented in literature and no definite conclusions can be taken with current knowledge. Artificial ovulation induction, potential changes in follicular and oocyte intracellular environments, extra-corporeal manipulation of gametes and embryos, the process of freezing and thawing, and embryo biopsies may increase risk for birth defects in children conceived by ART (Terada et al., 2000; Ertzeid and Storeng, 2001).

Large studies with robust methodologies have suggested that children born after ART have an increased risk of birth defects compared to naturally conceived children (Ooki, 2011). According to literature, risk of major malformations (conditions that cause functional impairment or require surgical correction) may be increased by 25% to 40% after IVF/ICSI (Rimm et al., 2004; Hansen et al., 2005).

In a recent meta-analysis, Wen et al. compared 124,468 children conceived by ART with spontaneously conceived children, and suggested a significantly increased risk of birth defects in the first group (relative risk = 1.37, 95% CI 1.26-1.48), with no increased risk for ICSI when compared with conventional IVF (Wen et al., 2012).

On the other hand, the recent evaluation of more than 15,000 children born after ART reinforced similar birth defect rates compared to naturally conceived children (Yan et al., 2011). Data comparing ART and naturally conceived children showed similar major birth defect rates after adjustment for maternal age, parity and ethnicity (Anthony et al., 2002), in agreement with previous reports (Loft et al. 1999; Bonduelle et al. 2002).

A large population study in Denmark compared congenital abnormality rates among naturally conceived and fertility treatment offspring from subfertile couples, and found no differences in overall prevalence of congenital malformations. In addition, this study indicates that parental factors such as increasing time to pregnancy (TTP) should be considerably associated with a greater risk of birth defects (Zhu et al., 2006).

In the prospective study of Seggers et al., at the age of 2 years, prevalence of minor anomalies (examples: ear tags, short stature, scholiosis, hemangioma) and those clinically relevant (examples: hernias that need surgical correction, hypospadia, cryptorchidism, club foot) were also similar for singletons born following controlled ovarian hyperstimulation or modified natural cycle for IVF/ICSI, or natural conception in subfertile couples. The authors demonstrated that abnormalities, especially those clinically relevant, were significantly associated with TTP (adjusted *odds ratio* = 1.20; 95% CI 1.02-1.4) (Seggers et al., 2012).

Finally, mounting evidence suggests that parental infertility may be an important independent risk factor for birth defects (Joffe and Li, 1994; Gray and Wu, 2000; Rimm et al., 2011).

Nevertheless, in the majority of studies, naturally conceiving mothers are significantly younger, more likely to be parous and more ethnically diverse than ART mothers, and attempts to stratify patients according to infertility history or paternal age, for example, are uncommon. This is why it would not be wrong to consider the risk of birth defects as being more associated with heredity than with ART themselves (Basatemur and Sutcliffe, 2008).

Chromosomal Abnormalities

Different studies have reported increased chromosomal abnormalities, especially *de novo*, ranging from 1.5% to 3.3% (Loft et al. 1999; Bonduelle et al. 2002; Jozwiak et al., 2004). Risk of chromosomal abnormalities among children conceived by ICSI is estimated to be 5% (Bonduelle et al. 2002) due to chromosomal aberrations in the parents. This percentage seems to be significantly higher than the expected value of 0.5% for the general population (Jacobs et al., 1992).

In a recent systematic review, authors investigated the occurrence of changes in the karyotypes of children conceived by IVF with sperm obtained by percutaneous aspiration (PESA), microsurgical epididymal aspiration (MESA) or testicular extraction (TESE), and found no association with augmented incidence of abnormal karyotype (Woldringh et al., 2009).

Epigenetic Inheritance

Classically associated with the modulation of the expression of a genotype into an unique phenotype, epigenetic inheritance is modernly referred to all mechanisms involved in the transfer of non-genetic information, as those that switch genes on and off, leading to mitotically and/or meiotically heritable changes in gene functions that do not imply modifications in DNA (Wu and Morris, 2001; Dupont et al., 2009). The more well-studied epigenetic mechanisms involve interplaying DNA methylation, RNA-mediated chromatin modifications, histone modifications and histone variants (van Montfoort et al., 2012).

Clinical relevance of the issue is based on the idea that any disturbance of the normal environment during gametogenesis, folliculogenesis and/or embryogenesis could evolve with undesirable misregulation in epigenetic inheritance (Dupont et al., 2009).

In spite of being more evident in mice than in humans (van Montfoort et al., 2012; de Waal et al., 2012), gene expression modifications heritable to forthcoming cell generations under epigenetic control have been described in children conceived *in vitro* (Katari et al., 2009). Such changes are suggested to be involved with imprinted genes, especially the Beckwith-Wiedemann syndrome (BWS) (Amor and Halliday, 2008; Ceelen et al., 2008b; Manipalviratn et al., 2009) and Angelmann syndrome (AS) (Lawrence and Moley, 2008), but a survey of more than 2,000 ART children showed that the absolute risk for disorders such as BWS and AS was less than 1% (Bowdin et al., 2007).

It has also been suggested that epigenetic effects may put IVF conceived children at greater risk to develop health problems in later life, like diabetes, obesity (Katari et al., 2009), cancer, coronary heart disease and stroke (Dupont et al., 2009).

According to Sato et al. (2007), ovarian stimulation with gonadotropins may be responsible for DNA methylation and disturbances in the expression of some imprinted genes in oocytes (Sato et al., 2007). The study of Ibala-Romdhane et al. (2011) analyzed *in vivo* matured human oocytes and found methylation disturbances to be more frequent than BWS after IVF. The authors observed significant hypomethylation of paternal alleles, which were attributed to unstable imprinting in the early stages of embryo development, and abnormal methylation of maternal alleles in arrested embryos. Conventional IVF did not differ from ICSI regarding methylation defects (Ibala-Romdhane et al., 2011).

Finally, the rarity of imprinting anomalies in the general population raise controversies and uncertainties, which means that one can not determine its true incidence in children conceived by IVF / ICSI.

Growth and Physical Health

Regarding growth of children, most studies have shown no differences between those conceived by ART and those conceived naturally. Basatemur et al. found similar weights and heights in the first 12 years of life of both groups (Basatemur et al., 2010), reinforcing previous data (Wennerholm et al., 1998; Brandes et al., 1992; Bonduelle et al., 2005; Ludwig et al., 2008; Belva et al., 2007; Knoester et al., 2008; Banerjee et al., 2008).

However, controversial findings were also published. In the study of Koivura et al., significantly lower weight was found among IVF children up to 3 years of age (Koivurova et al., 2003). Even height was demonstrated to differ between groups, but now it was found that

5 to 6 year-old children, born from IVF/ICSI, were taller than those from natural conception (Miles et al., 2007).

Bonduelle et al. described a higher probability of disease in children conceived by IVF/ICSI during their first 5 years (Bonduelle et al., 2005), among which prevail respiratory disorders and diarrhoea (Koivurova et al., 2003). However, most studies found no statistically significant differences concerning to chronic diseases between children conceived by ART or naturally, until 8 years of age (Place et al., 2003; Wennerhorm et al., 1998; Ludwig et al., 2009; Knoester et al., 2008).

Neurological Development

Middelburg et al. recently assessed outcomes of children conceived by IVF/ICSI in terms of neuromotor development, cognition, speech/language and behavior, and could not identify negative interference in developing the brain (Middelburg et al., 2008). Other prospective controlled studies found no difference in neurological outcomes among infants between 5-8 years born from ART and those conceived spontaneously (Bonduelle et al., 2004, Ludwig et al., 2008; Belva et al., 2007; Knoester et al., 2007a).

Evidence indicate moderately increased risk of epilepsy in children conceived by ART. Ericson et al. studied children between 1 and 11 years of age, and observed increased risk of hospitalization for epilepsy among those conceived by IVF (odds ratio 1.54, 95% CI 1.10-2.15). Statistically significant increased odds ratio (OR) were also observed for hospitalization in cases of cerebral palsy (OR 1.7, 95% CI 1.06-2.68), congenital malformation (OR 1.8, 95% CI 1.67-2.03), tumors (OR 1.6, 95% CI 1.16-2.13), asthma after one year of age (OR 1.4, 95% CI 1.2-1.56) or any infection (OR 1.4, 95% 1.29-1.44), but such excess were attributable to maternal subfertility (Ericson et al., 2002). TTP (Kallen et al., 2005) and prematurity (Sun et al., 2007) seem to be more associated with epilepsy than the reproductive treatment itself. Whereas events like cerebral palsy and epilepsy are rare. Studies of thousands of children would be required to achieve the statistical power needed to associate risks of these conditions to ART.

Psychosocial and Familiar Development

Literature is controversial on psychosocial and familiar development of children conceived by ART. Hahn revised psychosocial well-being of ART families and found no statistically significant differences regarding emotion, behavior, self-esteem or familiar perceptions among those children (Hahn, 2001). Also, Levy-Shiff et al. demonstrated similar intelligence quotients and cognitive performance between ART-conceived and naturally conceived children (Levy-Shiff et al. 1998).

As a matter of fact, other authors suggest that stress generated by infertility may conduct to dysfunctional parenting patterns and negative consequences for the child (Burns et al., 1990). Parents undergoing IVF commonly present low self esteem and feelings of incompetence, and may become overprotective or create unrealistic expectations in relation to their children (van Balen et al. 1998). Moreover, preterm infants are prone to develop behavioral disorders (Bhutta et al. 2002) and ART-conceived children have been described by teachers as more anxious, depressive and aggressive when compared to those naturally conceived (Levy-Shiff et al. 1998).

Finally, Williams et al. demonstrated an augmented incidence of autism among ICSI children (3,4%) when compared to general population (0,3%) (Williams et al. 2006), but Knoester et al. did not confirm such affirmative and found normal psychosocial behavior among ICSI children with 5 to 8 years of age (Knoester et al., 2007b).

References

Aboulghar, M., Evers, J. H., Al-Inany, H. Intravenous albumin for the preventing severe ovarian hyperstimulation syndrome: A Cochrane review. *Hum. Reprod.* 2002; 17:3027-32.

Aboulghar, M. Agonist and antagonist coast. *Fertil. Steril.* 2012; 97(3):523-6.

Abreu, L. G., Santana, L. F., Navarro, P. A. A. S., Reis, R. M., Ferriani, R. A., Moura, M. D. The pregnancy rate in women submitted to assisted reproduction techniques is lower after the age of 30 years. *Rev. Bras. Ginecol. Obstet.* 2006;28:32-7.

Adamson, G. D., de Mouzon, J., Lancaster, P., Nygren, K. G., Sullivan, E., Zegers-Hochschild, F. World collaborative report on in vitro fertilization, 2000. *Fertil. Steril.* 2006; 85: 1586-621.

Al-Inany, H. G., Youssef, M. A. F. M., Aboulghar, M., Broekmans, F., Sterrenburg, M., Smit, J., Abou-Setta, A. M. GnRH antagonists are safer than agonists: an update of a Cochrane review. *Hum. Reprod. Update* 2011; 17(4):435.

Alleyassin, A., Khademi, A., Aghahosseini, M., Safdarian, L., Badenoosh, B., Akbari, H. E. Comparison of success rates in the medical management of ectopic pregnancy with single-dose and multiple dose administration of methotrexate: a prospective, randomized clinical trial. *Fertil. Steril.* 2006;85:1661-6.

Amor, D. J., Halliday, J. A review of known imprinting syndromes and their association with assisted reproduction technologies. *Hum. Reprod.* 2008;23:2826–2834.

Andersen, A. N., Goossens, V., Ferraretti, A. P., Bhattacharya, S., Felberbaum, R., de Mouzon, J., Nygren, K. G., European, IVF-monitoring (EIM) Consortium; European Society of Human Reproduction and Embriology (ESHRE). Assisted reproductive technology in Europe, 2004. Results generated from European registers by ESHRE. *Hum. Reprod.* 2008; 23: 756-71.

Anthony, S., Buitendijk, S. E., Dorrepaal, C. A., Lindner, K., Braat, D. D., den Ouden, A. L. Congenital malformations in 4224 children conceived after IVF. *Hum. Reprod.* 2002;17(8):2089-95.

Banerjee, I., Shevlin, M., Taranissi, M., Thornhill, A., Abdalla, H., Ozturk, O., Barnes, J., Sutcliffe, A. Health of children conceived after preimplantation genetic diagnosis: a preliminary outcome study. *Reprod. Biomed. Online* 2008;16:376-81.

Basatemur, E., Sutcliffe, A. Follow-up of children born after ART. *Placenta* 2008;29 Suppl. B:135-40.

Basatemur, E., Shevlin, M., Sutcliffe, A. Growth of children conceived by IVF and ICSI up to 12 years of age. *Reprod. Biomed. Online* 2010;20:144-9.

Belva, F., Henriet, S., Liebaers, I., Van Steirteghem, A., Celestin-Westreich, S., Bonduelle, M. Medical outcome of 8-year-old singleton ICSI children (born > or = 32 weeks' gestation) and a spontaneously conceived comparison group. *Hum. Reprod.* 2007;22:506-15.

Bjercke, S., Tanbo, T., Dale, P. O., Mørkrid, L., Abyholm, T. Human chorionic gonadotrophin concentrations in early pregnancy after in-vitro fertilization. *Hum. Reprod.* 1999;14(6):1642-6.

Bonduelle, M., Liebaers, I., Deketelaere, V., Derde, M. P., Camus, M., Devroey, P., Van Steirteghem, A. Neonatal data on a cohort of 2889 infants born after ICSI (1991-1999) and of 2995 infants born after IVF (1983-1999). *Hum. Reprod.* 2002;17(3):671-94.

Bonduelle, M., Wennerholm, U. B., Loft, A., Tarlatzis, B. C., Peters, C., Henriet, S., Mau, C., Victorin-Cederquist, A., Van Steirteghem, A., Balaska, A., Emberson, J. R., Sutcliffe, A. G. A multi-centre cohort study of the physical health of 5-year-old children conceived after intracytoplasmic sperm injection, in vitro fertilization and natural conception. *Human Reprod.* 2005; 20:413-419.

Bonduelle, M., Bergh, C., Niklasson, A., Palermo, G. D., Wennerholm, U. B. Medical follow up study of 5-year-old ICSI children. *Reprod. Biomed. Online* 2004;9:91-101.

Bowdin, S., Allen, C., Kirby, G., Brueton, L., Afnan, M., Barratt, C., Kirkman-Brown, J., Harrison, R., Maher, E. R., Reardon, W. A survey of assisted reproductive technology births and imprinting disorders. *Hum. Reprod.* 2007;22(12):3237-40.

Brandes, J. M., Scher, A., Itzkovits, J., Thaler, I., Sarid, M., Gershoni-Baruch, R. Growth and development of children conceived by in vitro fertilization. *Pediatrics* 1992; 90:424-9.

BRASIL. Conselho Federal de Medicina – CFM. Resolução no 1.957, de 15 de dezembro de 2010. Diário Oficial da União, de 06 de janeiro de 2011; Seção I: 79.

Brewer, C., Acharya, S., Thake, F., Tang, T., Balen, A. Effect of metformin taken in the 'fresh' in vitro fertilization/intracytoplasmic sperm injection cycle upon subsequent frozen embryo replacement in women with polycystic ovary syndrome. *Hum. Fertil.* (Camb.) 2010;13(3):134-42.

Bhutta, A. T., Cleves, M. A., Casey, P. H., Cradock, M. M., Anand, K. J. Cognitive and behavioral outcomes of school-aged who were borned pre term: a meta-analysis. *JAMA* 2002;288:728-37.

Budev, M. M., Arroliga, A. C., Falcone, T. Ovarian hyperstimulation syndrome. *Crit. Care Med.* 2005;33(10 Suppl.):301-6.

Burns, L. H. An exploratory study of perceptions of parenting after infertility. *Family Systems medicine* 1990;8(2):177-189.

Carvalho, B. R., Cabral, I. O., Nakagava, H. M., Silva, A. A., Barbosa, A. C. P. Woman's age and ovarian response in ICSI cycles. *JBRA - Assisted Reproduction.* 2010;14(1):24-27.

Carvalho, B. R., Silva, A. A., Cabral, I. O., Gomes Sobrinho, D. B., Nakagava, H. M., Barbosa, A. C. P. Laboratory air quality upgrade from ISO class 7 to ISO class 5 improves ICSI outcomes in young infertile women. *JBRA - Assisted Reproductio*n. 2012.;16(1): 23-6.

Ceelen, M., van Weissenbruch, M. M., Vermeiden, J. P., van Leeuwen, F. E., Delemarre-van deWaal, H. A. Growth and development of children born after in vitro fertilization. *Fertil. Steril.* 2008;90:1662–1673.

Chen, S. U., Chen, R. J., Shieh, J. Y., Chou, C. H., Lin, C. W., Lu, H. F., et al.. Human chorionic gonadotropin up-regulates expression of myeloid cell leukemia-1 protein in human granulosa-lutein cells: implication of corpus luteum rescue and ovarian hyperstimulation syndrome. *J. Clin. Endocrinol. Metab.* 2010;95:3982e92.

Chung, K., Coutifaris, C., Chalian, R., Lin, K., Ratcliffe, S. J., Castelbaum, A. J., Freedman, M. F., Barnhart, K. Factors influencing adverse perinatal outcomes in pregnancies achieved through use of in vitro fertilization. *Fertil. Steril.* 2006;86:1634-41.

D'Angelo, A., Amso, N. Embryo freezing for preventing ovarian hyperstimulation syndrome. *Cochrane Database Syst. Rev.* 2007;18(3):1-22.

Davies, M. J., Moore, V. M., Willson, K. J., Van Essen, P., Priest, K., Scott, H., Haan, E. A., Chan, A. Reproductive technologies and the risk of birth defects. *N Engl. J. Med.* 2012;366(19):1803-13.

De Waal, E., Yamazaki, Y., Ingale, P., Bartolomei, M. S., Yanagimachi, R., McCarrey, J. R. Gonadotropin stimulation contributes to an increased incidence of epimutations in ICSI-derived mice. *Hum. Mol. Genet.* 2012 [Epub. ahead of print].

Delvigne, A. Symposium: Update on prediction and management of OHSS. Epidemiology of OHSS. *Reprod. Biomed. Online* 2009;19:8-13.

Delvigne, A., Rozenberg, S.: Epidemiology and prevention of ovarian hyperstimulation syndrome (OHSS): A review. *Human Reproduction Update* 2002; 8:559–577.

Dupont, C., Armant, D. A., Brenner, C. A. Epigenetics: definition, mechanisms and clinical perspective. *Semin. Reprod. Med.* 2009; 27(5): 351-357.

Elito Junior, J., Montenegro, N. A., Soares R. da C., Camano, L. Unruptured ectopic pregnancy: diagnosis and treatment. State of art. *Rev. Bras. Ginecol. Obstet.* 2008;30(3):149-59.

Ericson, A., Nygren, K. G., Olausson, P. O., Kallen, B. Hospital care utilization of infants born after IVF. *Hum. Reprod.* 2002;17:929–32.

Ertzeid, G., Storeng, R. The impact of ovarian stimulation on implantation and fetal development in mice. *Hum. Reprod.* 2001;16:221-5.

European Society of Human Reproduction and Embriology (ESHRE). ART fact sheet. URL: http://www.eshre.eu/ESHRE/English/Guidelines-Legal/ART-fact-sheet/page.aspx/1061. Accessed in 2012, July 23rd.

Fernandes, A. M. S., Ribeiro, L. P., Moraes, F. H., Meira, P. C., Sollero, C. A., Yamada, E. M. Prevalence of ectopic pregnancy liable to surgical treatment in a public hospital from 1995 through 2000. *Rev. Assoc. Med. Bras.* 2004; 50(4): 413-6.

Fernandez, H., Gervaise, A. Ectopic pregnancies after infertility treatment: modern diagnosis e therapeutic strategy. *Hum. Reprod. Update* 2004;10(6):503-13.

Gomez, R., Gonzalez-Izquierdo, M., Zimmermann, R. C., Novella-Maestre, E., Alonso-Muriel, I., Sanchez-Criado, J. Low-dose dopamine agonist administration blocks vascular endothelial growth factor (VEGF)-mediated vascular hyperpermeability without altering VEGF receptor 2 dependent luteal angiogenesis in a rat ovarian hyperstimulation model. *Endocrinology* 2006;147(11):5400–11.

Gray, R. H., Wu, L. Y. Subfertility and risk of spontaneous abortion. *Am. J. Public Health* 2000;90:1452-4.

Hahn, C. Review: Psychosocial well-being of parents and their children born after assisted reproduction. *Journal of Pediatric Psychology* 2001;26(8):525-38.

Hansen, M., Bower, C., Milne, E., de Klerk, N., Kurinczuk, J. J. Assisted reproductive technologies and the risk of birth defects – a systematic review. *Hum. Reprod.* 2005;20:328-38.

Humaidan, P., Quartarolo, J., Papanikolaou, E. G. Preventing ovarian hyperstimulation syndrome: guidance for the clinician. *Fertil. Steril.* 2010; 94(2):389-400.

Ibala-Romdhane, S., Al-Khtib, M., Khoueiry, R., Blachere, T., Guerin, J. F., Lefevre, A. Analysis of H19 methylation in control and abnormal human embryos, sperm and oocytes. *Eur. J. Hum. Genet.* 2011; 19(11): 1138-1143.

Jacobs, P. A., Browne, C., Gregson, N., Joyce, C., White, H. Estimates of the frequency of chromosome abnormalities detectable in unselected newborns using moderate levels of banding. *J. Med. Genet.* 1992;29(2):103-8.

Joffe, M., Li, Z. Association of time to pregnancy and the outcome of pregnancy. *Fertil. Steril.* 1994;62:71-5.

Jozwiak, E. A., Ulug, U., Mesut, A., Erden, H. F., Bahceci, M. Prenatal karyotypes of fetuses conceived by intracytoplasmic sperm injection. *Fertil. Steril.* 2004;82(3):628-33.

Jun, S. H., Milki, A. A. Ectopic Pregnancy rates with frozen compared with fresh blastocyst transfer. *Fertil. Steril.* 2007;88(3):629-31.

Kallen, B., Finnstrom, O., Nygren, K. G., Olausson, P. O. In vitro fertilization in Sweden: child morbidity including cancer risk. *Fertil. Steril.* 2005;84:605-10.

Katari, S., Turan, N., Bibikova, M., Erinle, O., Chalian, R., Foster, M., Gaughan, J. P., Coutifaris, C., Sapienza, C. DNA methylation and gene expression differences in children conceived in vitro or in vivo. *Hum. Mol. Genet.* 2009;18:3769-3778.

Klauser, C. K., May, W. L., Johnson, V. K., Cowan, B. D., Hines, R. S. Methotrexate for ectopic pregnancy: a randomized single dose compared with multiple dose. *Obstet. Gynaecol.* 2005;105:64S.

Klemetti, R., Sevón, T., Gissler, M., Hemminki, E. Health of Children Born as a Result of In Vitro Fertilization. *Pediatrics* 2006;118;1819-27.

Knoester, M., Vandenbroucke, J. P., Helmerhorst, F. M., van der Westerlaken, L. A., Walther, F. J., Veen, S. Matched follow-up study of 5–8 year old ICSI - singletons: comparison of their neuromotor development to IVF and naturally conceived singletons. *Hum. Reprod.* 2007a;22:1638–46.

Knoester, M., Helmerhorst, F. M., van der Westerlaken, Walther, F. J., Veen, S. Matched follow-up study of 5-8-year-old ICSI singletons: child behavior, parenting stress and child (health related) quality of life. *Human Reprod. Update* 2007b;22:3098-107.

Knoester, M., Helmerhorst, F. M., Vandenbroucke, J. P., van der Westerlaken, L. A.,Walther, F. J., Veen, S. Perinatal outcome, health, growth, and medical care utilization of 5- to 8-year-old intracytoplasmic sperm injection singletons. *Fertil. Steril.* 2008;89:1133–46.

Koivurova, S., Hartikainen, A. L., Sovio, U., Gissler, M., Hemminki, E., Jarvelin, R. Growth, psychomotor development and morbidity up to 3 years of age in children born after IVF. *Hum. Reprod.* 2003;18:2328-36.

Kol, S., Itskovitz-Eldor, J. Severe OHSS. Yes there is a strategy to prevent it! *Hum. Reprod.* 2000,15:2226-2227.

Kol, S., Homburg, R., Alsbjerg, B., Humaidan, P. The gonadotropin-releasing hormone antagonist protocol--the protocol of choice for the polycystic ovary syndrome patient undergoing controlled ovarian stimulation. *Acta Obstet. Gynecol. Scand.* 2012;91(6):643-7.

Lawrence, L. T. and Moley, K. H. Epigenetics and assisted reproductive technologies: human imprinting syndromes. *Semin. Reprod. Med.* 2008;26:143-52.

Lee, T. H., Liu, C. H., Huang, C. C., Wu, Y. L., Shih, Y. T., Ho, H. N., Yang, Y. S., Lee, M. S.: Serum anti -Müllerian hormone and estradiol levels as predictors of ovarian hyperstimulation syndrome in assisted reproduction technology cycles. *Hum. Reprod.* 2008, 23:160-167.

Levy-Shiff, R., Vakil, E., Dimitrovsky, L., Abramovitz, M., Shahar, N., Har-Even, D., Gross, S., Lerman, M., Levey, I., Sirota, L., Fish, B. Medical, cognitive, emotional and behavioral outcomes in school-age children conceived by in-vitro fertilization. *Journal of Clinical Child Psychology* 1998;27(3):320-9.

Lesny, P., Killick, S. R., Robinson, J., Maguiness, S. D. Transcervical embryo transfer as a risk factor for ectopic pregnancy. *Fertil. Steril.* 1999;72:305-309.

Loft, A., Petersen, K., Erb, K., Mikkelsen, A. L., Grinsted, J., Hald, F., et al.. A Danish national cohort of 730 infants born after intracytoplasmic sperm injection (ICSI) 1994-1997. *Hum. Reprod.* 1999;14(8):2143-8.

Ludwig, A. K., Katalinic, A., Thyen, U., Sutcliffe, A. G., Diedrich, K., Ludwig, M. Physical health at 5.5 years of age of term-born singletons after intracytoplasmic sperm injection: results of a prospective, controlled, single-blinded study. *Fertil. Steril.* 2009;91(1):115-24.

Luna, M., Grunfeld, L., Mukherjee, T., Sandler, B., Copperman, A. B. Moderately elevated levels of basal follicle-stimulating hormone in young patients predict low ovarian response, but should not be used to disqualify patients from attempting in vitro fertilization. *Fertil. Steril.* 2007;87:782-7.

Manipalviratn, S., DeCherney, A., Segars, J. Imprinting disorders and assisted reproductive technology. *Fertil. Steril.* 2009;91:305–315.

Mathur, R. S., Akande, V. A., Keay, S. D., Hunt, L. P., Jenkins, J. M.: Distinction between early and late ovarian hyperstimulation syndrome. *Fertil. Steril.* 2000, 73:901-907.

Middelburg, K. J., Heineman, M. J., Bos, A. F., Hadders-Algra, M. Neuromotor, cognitive, language and behavioural outcome in children born following IVF or ICSI - a systematic review. *Hum. Reprod. Update* 2008;14:219-31.

Miles, H. L., Hofman, P. L., Peek, J., Harris, M., Wilson, D., Robinson, E. M., Gluckman, P. D., Cutfield, W. S. In vitro fertilization improves childhood growth and metabolism. *J. Clin. Endocrinol. Metab.* 2007;92:3441-5.

Milki, A. A., Jun, S. H. Ectopic Pregnancy rates - Day 3 Versus Day 5 embryo transfer. A retrospective analysis. *BMC Pregnancy Childbirth* 2003;3(1):7.

Mol, F., Mol, B. W., Ankum, W. M., van der Veen, F., Hajenius, P. J. Current evidence on surgery, systemic methotrexate and expectant management in the treatment of tubal ectopic pregnancy: a systematic review and meta-analysis. *Hum. Reprod. Update* 2008;14(4):309-19.

Mullin, C., Berkeley, A. S., Grifo, J. A. Supernumerary Blastocyst Cryopreservation: A key Prognostic Indicator for Patients Opting for an Elective Single Blastocyst Transfer (eSBT). *J. Assist. Reprod. Genet.* 2012 [Epub. ahead of print].

Nelson, S. M., Lawlor, D. A. (2011) Predicting Live Birth, Preterm Delivery, and Low Birth Weight in Infants Born from In Vitro Fertilisation: A Prospective Study of 144,018 Treatment Cycles. *PLoS Med.* 8(1): e1000386. doi:10.1371/journal.pmed.1000386.

Ooki, S. Birth Defects in Singleton versus Multiple ART Births in Japan (2004-2008). *J. Pregnancy.* 2011;2011:285706.

Palomba, S., Falbo, A., Carrillo, L., Villani, M. T., Orio, F., Russo, T., Di Cello, A., Cappiello, F., Capasso, S., Tolino, A., Colao, A., Mastrantonio, P., La Sala, G. B., Zullo, F., Cittadini, E.; METformin in High Responder Italian Group. Metformin reduces risk of ovarian hyperstimulation syndrome in patients with polycystic ovary syndrome during gonadotropin-stimulated in vitro fertilization cycles: a randomized, controlled trial. *Fertil. Steril.* 2011 Dec.;96(6):1384-1390.e4. Epub. 2011 Oct. 7.

Papanikolaou, E. G., Pozzobon, C., Kolibianakis, E. M., Camus, M., Tournaye, H., Fatemi, H. M., van Steirteghem, A., Devroey, P. Incidence and prediction of ovarian hyperstimulation syndrome in women undergoing gonadotropin releasing hormone antagonist in vitro fertilization cycles. *Fertil. Steril.* 2006;85(1):120-9.

Papanikolaou, et al..: New algorithm for OHSS prevention. *Reproductive Biology and Endocrinology* 2011 9:147.

Place, I., Englert, Y. A prospective longitudinal study of the physical, psychomotor, and intellectual development of singleton children up to 5 years who were conceived by intracytoplasmic sperm injection compared with children conceived spontaneously and by in vitro fertilization. *Fertil. Steril.* 2003;80: 1388–97.

Pinborg, A., Lidegaard, O., la Cour Freiesleben, N., Andersen, A. N. Consequences of vanishing twins in IVF/ICSI pregnancies. *Hum. Reprod.* 2005;20:2821-9.

Poikkeus, P., Hiilesmaa, V., Tiitinen, A. Serum HCG 12 days after embryo transfer in predicting pregnancy outcome. *Hum. Reprod.* 2002;17(7):1901-5.

Rimm, A. A., Katayama, A. C., Diaz, M., Katayama, K. P. A meta-analysis of controlled studies comparing major malformation rates in IVF and ICSI infants with naturally conceived children. *J. Assist. Reprod. Genet.* 2004;21(12):437-43.

Rimm, A. A., Katayama, A. C., Katayama, K. P. A meta-analysis of the impact of IVF and ICSI on major malformations after adjusting for the effect of subfertility. *J. Assist. Reprod. Genet.* 2011;28(8):699-705.

Sapienza, C. DNA methylation and gene expression differences in children conceived in vitro or in vivo. *Hum. Mol. Genetic* 2009; 18(20): 3769-3778.

Sato, A., Otsu, E., Negishi, H., Utsunomiya, T., and Arime, T. Aberrant DNA methylation of imprinted loci in superovulated oocytes. *Hum. Reprod.* 2007;22:26-35.

Schieve, L. A., Peterson, H. B., Meikle, S. F., Jeng, G., Danel, I., Burnett, N. M., Wilcox, L. S. Live-birth rates and multiple-birth risk using in vitro fertilization. *JAMA* 1999;282(19):1832-8.

Seggers, J., Haadsma, M. L., Bos, A. F., Heineman, M. J., Keating, P., Middelburg, K. J., van Hoften, J. C., Veenstra-Knol, H. E., Kok, J. H., Cobben, J. M., Hadders-Algra, M. Dysmorphic features in 2-year-old IVF/ICSI offspring. *Early Hum. Dev.* 2012 [Epub. ahead of print].

Soares, S. R. Etiology of OHSS and use of dopamine agonists. *Fertil. Steril.* 2012;97(3):517-22.

Society for Assisted Reproductive Technology and the American Society for Reproductive Medicine. Assisted reproductive technology in the United States: 2001 results generated from the American Society for Reproductive Medicine/Society for Assisted Reproductive Technology registry. *Fertil. Steril.* 2007;87:1253-66.

Steptoe, P. C., Edwards, R. G. Reimplantation of a human embryo with subsequent tubal pregnancy. *Lancet* 1976;(7965);728-9.

Sun, Y., Vestergaard, M., Christensen, J., Zhu, J. L., Bech, B. H., Olsen, J. Epilepsy and febrile seizures in children of treated and untreated subfertile couples. *Hum. Reprod.* 2007;22:215-20.

Tehraninejad, E. S., Hafezi, M., Arabipoor, A., Aziminekoo, E., Chehrazi, M., Bahmanabadi, A. Comparison of cabergoline and intravenous albumin in the prevention of ovarian hyperstimulation syndrome: a randomized clinical trial. *J. Assist. Reprod. Genet.* 2012;29:259-64.

Terada, Y., Luetjens, C. M., Sutovsky, P., Schatten, G. Atypical decondensation of the sperm nucleus, delayed replication of the male genome, and sex chromosome positioning following intracytoplasmic human sperm injection (ICSI) into golden hamster eggs: does ICSI itself introduce chromosomal anomalies? *Fertil. Steril.* 2000;74:454-60.

The Practice Committee of the American Society for Reproductive Medicine. Ovarian hyperstimulation syndrome. *Fertil. Steril.* 2008a; 90:S188–93.

The Practice Committee of the American Society for Reproductive Medicine. The role of tubal reconstructive surgery in the era of assisted reproductive technologies. *Fertil. Steril.* 2008b;90:S250-3.

The Practice Committee of the American Society for Reproductive Medicine. Medical treatment of ectopic pregnancy. *Fertil. Steril.* 2008c; 90:S206–12.

Van Balen, F. Development of IVF children. *Developmental Review* 1998;18(1):30-46.

Van Montfoort, A. P. A., Hanssen, L. L. P., de Sutter, P., Viville, S., Geraedts, J. P. M., de Boer, P. Assisted reproduction treatment and epigenetic inheritance. *Hum. Reprod. Update* 2012;18(2):171-97.

Veleva, Z., Karinen, P., Tomas, C., Tapanainen, J. S., Martikainen, H. Elective single embryo transfer with cryopreservation improves the outcome and diminishes the costs of IVF/ICSI. *Hum. Reprod.* 2009;24(7):1632-9.

Wen, J., Jiang, J., Ding, C., Dai, J., Liu, Y., Xia, Y., Liu, J., Hu, Z. Birth defects in children conceived by in vitro fertilization and intracytoplasmic sperm injection: a meta-analysis. *Fertil. Steril.* 2012;97(6):1331-7.

Wennerholm, U. B., Albertsson-Wikland, K., Bergh, C., Hamberger, L., Niklasson, A., Nisson, L., Thiringer, K., Wennergren, M., Wikland, M., Borres, M. P. Postnatal growth and health in children born after cryopreservation as embryos. *Lancet* 1998;351:1085-90.

Williams, J. G., Higgins, J. P., Brayne, C. E. Systematic review of prevalence studies of autism spectrum discorders. *Arch. Dis. Child* 2006;91:8-15.

Woldringh, G. H., Besselink, D. E., Tillema, A. H., Hendriks, J. C., Kremer, J. A. Karyotyping, congenital anomalies and follow-up of children after intracytoplasmic sperm injection with non-ejaculated sperm: a systematic review. *Hum. Reprod. Update* 2010;16(1):12-9.

Wright, V. C., Chang, J., Jeng, G., Macaluso, M. Assisted reproductive technology surveillance – United States, 2005. *MMWR Surveill. Summ.* 2008; 57:1-23.

Wu, Ct., Morris, J. R. Genes, genetics, and epigenetics: a correspondence. *Science* 2001;293(5532): 1103–1105.

Yan, J., Huang, G., Sun, Y., Zhao, X., Chen, S., Zou, S., Hao, C., Quan, S., Chen, Z. J. Birth defects after assisted reproductive technologies in China: analysis of 15,405 offspring in seven centers (2004 to 2008). *Fertil. Steril.* 2011;95(1):458-60.

Youssef, M. A. F. M., van Wely, M., Hassan, M. A., Al-Inany, H. G., Mochtar, M., Khattab, S., van der Veen, F. Can dopamine agonists reduce the incidence and severity of OHSS in IVF/ICSI treatment cycles? A systematic review and meta-analysis. *Hum. Reprod. Update* 2010;16:459-66.

Youssef, M. A. F. M., Al-Inany, H. G., Evers, J., Aboulghar, M. Intra-venous fluids for the prevention of severe ovarian hyperstimulation syndrome. *Cochrane Database Syst. Rev.* 2012; 1:

Zegers-Hochschild, F., Schwarze, J. E., Galdames, V. (Eds). Red Latinoamericana de Reproducción Asistida. Registro Latinoamericano de Reproducción Asistida. 2008. URL: http:// www.redlara.com/imagens/arq/ 2008_ registro%202008.pdf. Accessed in July 23rd, 2012.

Zhu, J. L., Basso, O., Obel, C., Bille, C., Olsen, J. Infertility, infertility treatment, and congenital malformations: Danish national birth cohort. *BMJ.* 2006 Sep. 30;333(7570):679.

In: Infertility
Editors: R. Nascimento and H. V. Boas
ISBN: 978-1-62257-909-9

Chapter 3

The Impact of Follicular Fluid Components and Embryo-endometrial Cross-talk on the Oocyte Quality or Embryo Viability: Search for New Biomarkers

M. Králíčková[1,2]***, M. Čedíková***[1,3]***, P. Pitule***[1,3]***, P. Šíma***[4]
and V. Větvička[5,*]
[1]Department of Histology and Embryology, Faculty of Medicine, Charles University, Plzen, Czech Republic
[2]Department of Obstetrics and Gynecology, University Hospital, Faculty of Medicine, Charles University, Plzen, Czech Republic
[3]Biomedical Centre, Faculty of Medicine in Plzen, Charles University, Plzen, Czech Republic
[4]Department of Immunology and Gnotobiology, Institute of Microbiology, Czech Academy of Sciences, Prague, Czech Republic
[5]University of Louisville, Department of Pathology, Louisville, KY, US

Abstract

To overcome the still insufficient implantation rate following *in vitro* fertilization (IVF) in humans, more than two embryos are commonly replaced which potentially leads to a high number of multiple pregnancies with associated risks such as low birth weight. The solution for avoiding multiple pregnancies could be optimalization of embryo selection and single embryo transfer.

The traditional systems for assessing gamete and embryo viability have limited ability to accurately select those with the best developmental potential. Morphological

[*] Correspondence to: Vaclav Vetvicka, University of Louisville, Department of Pathology, 511 S. Floyd, Louisville, KY 40202, U.S.A. email: vaclav.vetvicka@louisville.edu.

evaluation remains the primary method of oocyte and embryo assessment during IVF cycles. However, its modest predictive power and inherent inter- and intra-observer variability limits its clinical value. Prolonged embryo culture to blastocyst stage was introduced as a possible strategy for selecting the best embryos but the extended period of *in vitro* culture may have its side effects.

Successful embryo implantation requires accurate temporal regulation of maternal immune functions to accommodate a semi-allogeneic embryo. To prepare the immunological tolerance at the beginning of implantation, the precise temporal regulations between the immune and endocrine components are required. Our review will focus on molecules of embryo-endometrial cross-talk that are engaged in regulation of the embryo implantation, and on selected follicular fluid components that might play a role in developmental/embryogenic potential of the oocyte.

The review will also discuss advances in the understanding of the regulation of fertility that has been made during last 15 years with the production of over 400 mutant mouse models with a reproductive phenotype. Indeed, the past few years have witnessed a virtual explosion in the identification of gene mutations or polymorphisms that cause or are linked to human infertility and that are inherited in a polygenic/multifactorial fashion.

The aim of this review is to point out two recent trends in reproductive medicine - the search for potentially useful biomarkers for improvement of pregnancy rates after the assisted reproduction techniques (ART); and the importance of homeostasis that makes spontaneous conception possible. Especially in diagnoses like the endometriosis, the causes of infertility remains not fully understood and the best option for these patients is a return to the balance that enables the spontaneous conception.

Introduction

Since the first successful *in vitro* fertilization (IVF) in humans and the birth of Louise Joy Brown, the world's first test-tube baby in 1978, the number of patients using Assisted Reproductive Technologies (ART) has increased tremendously. ART have increased in number, their spectrum has widened and, of course, their efficiency is increasing. But ART are not efficient enough yet and even today, many women seeking medical treatment for infertility never give birth to a child.

Successful implantation requires a functionally normal, viable embryo (or embryos) at the blastocyst stage and a receptive endometrium. The embryo - endometrium cross-talk is highly regulated. Numerous molecules are taking part, organized in a hierarchized cascade of events initiated by steroid hormones and mediated by a row of cytokines, growth factors and integrins that determine establishment of a timely dialogue between endometrium and blastocyst.

Current ART as well as most of present investigative attention in the field of infertility are devoted mainly to the embryo or the endometrium. For the enhancement of ART efficiency, it is necessary to pay more investigative effort to the marginalized topic, the role of molecular vectors transferring the cross-talk signals between the maternal uterine tissues and trophoblast and subsequently to transfer new findings in two directions – to identify potential biomarkers for prediction of the success of infertility treatment and to enable new ways in the infertility treatment by returning the homeostasis and making the spontaneous conception possible again.

Assisted Reproductive Technologies - On the Search of "Positive" and "Negative" Predictive Markers

Infertility affects 10-15% of couples at reproductive age. At present, a strong demand for assistance in resolving this problem exists, but the implantation and pregnancy rates following IVF are still not sufficient [1, 2]. To increase the success of the treatment, more than two embryos are commonly replaced, which might potentially result in high number of multiple pregnancies with associated elevated risks such as low birth weight. Possible solution for avoiding multiple pregnancies could be optimalization of embryo selection and subsequent single embryo transfer.

Morphological criteria remains the primary method of the oocyte and embryo assessment during IVF cycles, but its modest predictive power and inherent inter- and intra-observer variability limits its value [3]. Prolonged embryo culture to blastocyst stage was introduced as a possible strategy for selecting the best embryos. Unfortunately, the method has its limits in increasing the rates and the extended period of *in vitro* culture may have its side effects – e. g. predispose the embryo to phenomenon such as 'large offspring syndrome,' which is probably linked to altered gene expression, particularly of imprinted genes [4].

It is supposed that evaluation criteria should be changed by adding the detection of certain molecular markers (either in follicular fluid, blood or embryo culture media) that will have a predictive value. In the follicular fluid, various molecules have already been proved to be reliable in predicting the oocyte quality or even embryo viability. These have the potential to be used during infertility treatment as "positive predictive markers." Results obtained by our group [5, 6] demonstrated that *lif* gene mutations coincide with infertility but do not influence the infertility treatment outcome in general, only in the presence of certain other factors or diagnosis, e.g. endometriosis, therefore serving as "negative predictive markers." Both approaches could be combined and lead to individualization of the therapy, which is highly desirable way of approach.

What is the Role of Genetic Alterations in Infertility?

Pivotal information has been derived for a host of rare genetic disorders. Unfortunately, in the common causes of female infertility, the progress has been much slower. Many infertile couples continue to be diagnosed as idiopathic infertility or given descriptive diagnoses not providing a real cause for their reproductive defect.

Important advances in the understanding of the treatment of infertility have been made during last 15 years, with the production of over 400 mutant mouse models with a reproductive phenotype (for review see [7-9]). Indeed, the past years have witnessed a virtual explosion in the identification of genetic mutations or polymorphisms that cause or are linked to human infertility and that are inherited in a polygenic/multifactorial fashion (for review see [10]). Nevertheless, translation of these findings to the clinical practice remains agonizingly slow.

There are three necessary conditions for successful embryo implantation – the viable embryo, the receptive endometrium, and their mutual molecular cross-talk [11]. Under the influence of steroid hormones and paracrine signals from the developing embryo, the endometrium becomes receptive for only a limited period of time. The receptive state is characterized by the expression of particular genes that allow the refractory endometrium to respond to the embryo and permit attachment.

Numerous studies in mice have suggested the importance of different cytokines produced by both embryo and maternal tissue [12, 13] and participating in the cross-talk between the implanting blastocyst and the endometrium [14]. The presence of complex network of cytokines and their overlapping biological activities means that alteration of one cytokine is likely to affect others, making studies of their role in implantation failure extremely difficult.

p53 – A New Player in Reproduction Regulation

The p53 (OMIM*191170) is a key tumor suppressor. Its function is lost in many types of cancers, either by mutation or by excessive negative regulation (for review see [15]). Since 2002, several groups have identified the existence of several p53 isoforms and have demonstrated their roles in modulation of p53 suppressive activity in cancer (for review see [16]). However, little is known about p53's normal physiological function. Recently, it has been shown that p53 is important in reproduction in a gender-specific manner [17]. Significant decreases in embryonic implantation, pregnancy rate and litter size were observed in mating with $p53^{-/-}$ female mice but not with $p53^{-/-}$ male mice. The gene encoding leukemia inhibitory factor (LIF) was identified as a p53-regulated gene that functions as the downstream mediator of this effect. p53 can regulate both basal and inducible transcription of LIF and loss of p53 decreased both the level and function of LIF in uterus. Lower LIF levels were observed in the uterus of $p53^{-/-}$ mice than in those of $p53^{+/+}$ mice, particularly at day 4 of pregnancy when transiently induced high levels of LIF were crucial for embryonic implantation [18, 19]. This observation probably accounts for the impaired implantation of embryos in $p53^{-/-}$ female mice. Administration of LIF to pregnant $p53^{-/-}$ mice restored maternal reproduction by improving implantation. These results clearly confirm function for p53 in maternal reproduction through the regulation of LIF [20, 21].

Evidence is accumulating that p53 may have a similar function in humans - an association has been reported between women carrying the p53 codon 72 mutation (a proline to arginine change) and recurrent implantation failure [21]. In addition, the p53 gene was suggested to be a candidate gene for endometriosis [22]. The p53 pathway is therefore the subject of intense research trying to identify its role in both cancer and infertility.

The Role of LIF in Embryo Implantation

The LIF is a pluripotent cytokine that plays a central role in the control of the embryo implantation. LIF (OMIM*159540) is a secreted glycoprotein first described as a factor inducing the differentiation of myeloid leukemic M1 cells into macrophages [23]. An important role for LIF in implantation was shown in LIF knockout mice, where embryo implantation did not occur [24]. In endometrium of healthy women, LIF and LIF mRNA are expressed throughout the menstrual cycle with a striking increase in the midsecretory phase, coinciding with a supposed window of implantation. Binding of LIF to LIF receptor (LIFR) activates signal transduction pathways [25]. Human blastocysts express mRNAs for LIFR participating actively in establishing contact with the endometrium. In the endometrium, LIFR are expressed in the epithelium throughout the cycle with strong increase in the midsecretory phase. Endometrium of infertile women produces significantly less LIF during the period of receptivity [26]. In addition, LIF is detected in uterine flushing, and its level is significantly lower in women with idiopathic infertility. Likewise, endometrial explants derived from women with idiopathic infertility showed reduced levels of LIF secretion (for review see [27-29]).

The first report of *lif* gene mutations in human searched for mutations in 74 non-selected nulligravid infertile women and identified three point mutations. Two of them were G to A transitions located in exon 3 at the positions 3400 and 3424 of the *lif* gene that lead to an amino acid exchanges (valine 64 methionine and alanine 72 threonine) in the regions corresponding to AB loop of the LIF protein. The AB loop seems to be highly important for interaction with the LIFR, so that the mutation causing the amino acid exchange within the region could result in reduced biological activity of the LIF protein. The third mutation, the C to A transition at position 715, was located in the regulatory region, 6 bp from the start codon of the LIF gene. It was hypothesized that this mutation could lead to transcription abnormalities and result in the decreased LIF expression [30].

The second report of *lif* gene mutations in infertile women focused on patients with recurrent failure of IVF or intracytoplasmatic sperm injection, defined as three or more embryo transfers, and on women diagnosed with unexplained infertility for at least two years. The previously described G to A transition at the position 3400 and the G to A transition at position 3441 were identified in nulligravid women with unexplained infertility. The G to T transition at the position 3453 was identified in a nulligravid woman with more then three failure of IVF. Both newly described transitions, at the position 3453 and 3441, did not cause the protein structure alterations. The only one woman with the heterozygous potentially functional mutation at position 3400 conceived after IVF treatment. From these results, the authors concluded that the second allele of the *lif* gene, stimulated hormonally during superovulated cycle, might compensate the defect [31]. Their hypothesis was supported by another study, which demonstrated that LIF on luminal epithelium enhances the expression of a subset of progesterone-regulated genes [25].

In our studies 15 positive samples were identified in exon 3.2 in the group of infertile women (n=176) [5, 6]. All samples showed an alteration in DNA sequence that was identical to previously described potentially functional *lif* gene point mutation, the G to A transition at the position 3400. Out of the 15 infertile women, the group A was made up of women with diagnoses that are frequently accompanied by changes in humoral and cell mediated immunity - idiopathic infertility and endometriosis (n=7). Group B was comprised of patients with polycystic ovary syndrome, andrological factor, tubal factor and hyperprolactinemia (n=8). The control group was comprised of 136 infertile women with no *lif* gene mutation diagnosed with idiopathic infertility and endometriosis (n=37) (group C) and patients with polycystic ovary syndrome, tubal and andrological factor (n=99) (group D). Seven of the mutation-positive patients were successfully treated by IVF, but in this group there was no diagnosis of idiopathic infertility and only one of endometriosis, meaning that there is a statistically significant difference in the pregnancy rates between groups A and B, but no statistically significant difference when comparing patients with the *lif* gene mutation (group A+B) to no *lif* gene mutation (group C+D). These results suggest that the idiopathic infertility and endometriosis have a negative impact on the outcome of IVF treatment in mutation-positive women [6].

The Role of IL-11 in Endometrial Decidualisation

Interleukin 11 (IL-11) (OMIM*147681) is essential for murine implantation and signals *via* intracellular phosphorylation of STAT3 in the endometrium similar to LIF [32]. Both molecules are present in the endometrium of women during the receptive window. IL-11 expression is critically important during decidualization in the human endometrium and its aberrant regulation may be associated with some types of infertility [33]. Reduced endometrial pSTAT3 and IL-11 levels were shown in some women with idiopathic infertility [34] and in some endometriotic patients [35].

The Oocyte – Another Key Player in the Success of Implantation

The oocyte quality profoundly affects fertilization and subsequent embryo development driving the continued search for reliable predictors of oocyte developmental competence. Traditional methods for the evaluation of oocyte quality are based on morphological classification of the follicle, cumulus-oocyte complex, polar body and/or meiotic spindle (for review see [36]). Several intrinsic (such as mitochondrial status and glucose-6-phosphate dehydrogenase 1 activity) and extrinsic markers (such as apoptosis of follicular cells, levels of the transforming growth factor-beta superfamily, anti-müllerian hormone, inhibin B, granulocyte colony stimulating factor, macrophage colony stimulating factor and vascular endothelial growth factor in follicular fluid (FF)) have also been reported as useful indicators of oocyte competence and embryo quality [37-46]. In some cases, the controversy about the role of an individual marker remains – e.g. in the question whether LIF or leptin in FF can predict the oocyte quality or outcome of IVF, there were various studies done with contradictory results [47-49].

Oxidative Stress in Follicular Fluid (FF) – A Field for Search of Valid Biomarkers?

Oxidative stress is defined as an increased intracellular concentration of the reactive oxygen species (ROS) in a steady-state condition. The possibility that ROS and oxygen radicals might be involved in human reproduction was suggested nearly 80 years ago [50]. Their pathological effects result from damage to lipids (particularly in the cell membrane), nucleic acids, proteins and other cellular materials [51]. *In vivo*, the damaging effects of oxygen radicals are usually prevented or limited by endogenous antioxidants or scavengers of free radicals. These include enzymes such as superoxide dismutase, catalase and selenium-dependent glutathione peroxidase as well as lipid- and water-soluble antioxidants such as vitamins C, E and uric acid [52]. Ho et al. [53] and Matzuk et al. [54] reported decreased litter size and number of litters per month in female homozygous mutant mice lacking superoxide dismutase.

Proteome analysis of human follicular fluid from 25 normo-ovulatory women undergoing assisted reproduction techniques due to a male infertility factor (that means that they are fully fertile) identified several important antioxidant enzymes; i.e., catalase, superoxide dismutase, glutathione transferase, paraoxonase, heat shock protein 27 and protein disulfide isomerase. This indicates that during maturation the human follicle is well protected against toxic injury caused by oxidative stress [55].

Some findings suggest that cumulus cells may have a critical role in protecting oocytes against oxidative stress-induced apoptosis through the increase of glutathione content in oocytes [56]. Oxidative stress has an impact on the production of granulosa cell steroid hormones (estradiol in particular), which are important predictors of ovarian response. The positive association between FF estradiol and total antioxidant capacity (TAC) suggests that estradiol may play a role in the ovarian antioxidant-oxidant balance [57].

Individual FF analysis (from separate follicles) showed that ROS levels in FF participates in embryo formation and quality [58]. Both lipid peroxidation (LPO) and TAC levels were positively correlated with the pregnancy rate. LPO is a good marker of metabolic activity within the follicle, and some amounts may be necessary to establish a pregnancy [59-62]. Malondialdehyde can be used as another marker of oxidative stress and also in predicting assisted reproductive techniques outcome [63].

Although there was no significant relationship between plasma and/or FF TAC and the underlying etiology of infertility [57], the oxidative stress is engaged in pathophysiology of many of them. For example, the ROS action is one of the mechanisms responsible for the embryotoxicity of hydrosalpingeal fluid and for the decreased quality of oocytes and embryos of endometriosis patients [64]. Decreased levels of SeGPx were confirmed in FF of women with idiopathic infertility [65, 66].

The age-related decline of the success in IVF is largely attributable to a progressive decline of ovarian oocyte quality and quantity which can be at least partially caused by the age-related increase in free radical activity [67, 68]. It was confirmed that active smoking affects the pro-oxidant/antioxidant balance inside the pre-ovulatory ovarian follicle by inducing intrafollicular oxidative stress impairing folliculogenesis [69] especially by accelerated follicular depletion [70].

Detrimental effects of oxygen-derived free radicals on embryos during culture have been demonstrated in several species [71, 72]. Yang et al. [73] found higher levels of hydrogen peroxide in fragmented compared with non-fragmented human embryos and unfertilized oocytes, whilst Paszkowski and Clarke [66] reported increased antioxidant consumption (suggesting increased ROS activity) during incubation of poor quality embryos.

Infertility in Endometriosis Patients

Endometriosis is a common gynecological problem of reproductive-age women, and despite the increasing evidence proving genetic component to this disease, its basic etiology remains unclear.It is likely that it is a polygenic/multifactorial disease caused by an interaction between multiple genes [74]. The association between endometriosis and infertility is complex. There are four principle factors that contribute to subfertility - impaired folliculogenesis, decreased fertilization, inflammatory factors in follicular, peritoneal and reproductive tract fluid, and implantation defects [75, 76]. Nevertheless, in the absence of tubal distortion, spontaneous conception remains possible. That means that the optimal choice for endometriosis patients is to be treated and then to get pregnant after spontaneous conception.

Endometriosis in reproductive-age women is associated with various immunopathologies - there are changes in both cell-mediated and humoral immunity and these changes seem to play a crucial role in allowing endometriosis implants to persist and progress [77].

Many various cytokines are present in the peritoneal fluid. They are produced by a variety of cells including mesothelial cells, leukocytes and ectopic endometrial cells. Their increased levels might to promote implantation and growth of ectopic endometrium by inducing proliferation and angiogenesis [78, 79].

The peritoneal fluid of women with endometriosis contains increased numbers of cells which facilitate rather than inhibit the development of endometriosis. Macrophages that would be expected to clear endometrial cells from the peritoneal cavity appear to enhance their proliferation by secreting growth factors and cytokines [77, 80]. Nevertheless, the exact immunological mechanisms that support persistence and proliferation of ectopic endometrial implants within the peritoneal cavity remain unknown.

The observation that natural killer (NK) cell activity is abnormally low in endometriosis patients has lead to a hypothesis that the inhibition of NK and cytotoxic T-cell function is one of the key mechanisms of pathogenesis [81].

The reports about the role of LIF in the infertility of endometriosis patients are rather conflicting. In patients with endometriosis the LIF staining intensity in uterine epithelium was studied. Staining intensity of LIF was evaluated using semi-quantitative immunohistochemistry scores and immunoreactive LIF was present predominantly in glandular epithelium, while luminal epithelium showed patchy staining. LIF staining intensity in glandular epithelium was significantly lower in endometriosis and the results suggested that reduced endometrial LIF contributes to infertility in some endometriotic women [35].

In the mouse model, expression of LIF in endometrium peaked at the time of implantation and was reduced by injections of human peritoneal fluid from infertile patients with endometriosis. PF from women with endometriosis has a detrimental effect on embryo implantation, perhaps by adversely affecting LIF expression as well as uterine receptivity [82]. On the other hand, in the uterine flushings and endometrial samples from 7 to 9 days after ovulation no statistically significant differences in levels of LIF between endometriosis patients and controls were found. The authors concluded that there is no receptivity defect with regard to LIF secretion by eutopic endometrium in infertile women with endometriosis [83].

Role of NK Cells in Endometriosis and Infertility in General

Large populations of macrophages and uterine-specific (NK) cells infiltrate the implantation site, and arebelieved to be important modulators of trophoblast invasion and decidualization [84-86]. However, our knowledge regarding selective recruitment of leukocyte subtypes is not complete. Adequacy of the endometrium for fertility has been classically investigated by histologic evaluation of a mid-late luteal phase biopsy. Recent studies demonstrate histologically normal, but biochemically abnormal, endometrium during the window of implantation in some women with endometriosis [87]. Such evidence continues to reinforce the hypothesis that endometrium from some women with endometriosis might be dysfunctional. The reduced endometrial receptivity seems to account for the reduction in cycle fecundity [88].

Increased CD158a$^+$ NK cells in peripheral blood and peritoneal fluid indicates decreased NK cell cytotoxicity [89]. The percentage of these cells in blood as well as in perotoneal fluid is significantly higher in women with than without endometriosis [90]. These properties of NK cells (as well as macrophages) in women with endometriosis promote immunotolerance to implanted tissue in the peritoneal environment [90]. According the present knowledge, NK cells and their number as well as their low activity in endometriosis is mediated by cytokines and by HLA-G [91]. LIF is one of the cytokines that were shown to regulate NK cells. The *lif* gene knockout mice have doubled the percentage of NK cells in endometrium compared to wild-type mice at the time of implantation window, indicating that LIF restricts the migration of NK cells to the uterus [93]. Nevertheless, the mechanisms involved in homing of mouse uterine NK cell precursors to the uterus regulated by LIF are not fully understood yet. Strong expression of LIF mRNA was detected in decidual leukocytes, which are abundant at the implantation site. Extravillous trophoblast invading the maternal decidua expresses LIFR as it moves past decidual leukocytes, which express LIF mRNA. Although its effects on trophoblast are not clear, LIF appears to mediate interactions between maternal decidual leukocytes and invading trophoblast [94, 95]. LIF may also play a critical role in controlling angiogenesis in the placental villi, since human fetal endothelial cells express LIFR, and mice lacking a functional LIF receptor gene show altered vascular development in the placenta [96-98].

Various cytokines have already been suggested and some of them (such as TNF-binding protein-1 and IL-12) have already been proven to be effective in reducing endometriotic lesions in animal models, while pentoxifylline and INF-alpha 2b have shown encouraging results in clinical studies [99]. HLA-G is expressed by endometriotic glandular epithelium, but not by eutopic endometrium. Differential expression of HLA-G suggests that peritoneal inflammation or cellular stress may up-regulate mechanisms to promote ectopic endometrial survival [100].

There is a need for immunological diagnostics in the group of patients with unexplained infertility and endometriosis. It was proven that these patients suffer by various immunologic disturbances, some of the endometriosis patients are even at higher risk than the general female population of developing autoimmune and atopic disorders as well as breast and other cancers (for review see [101].

Conclusion

Present progress in various techniques gives researchers options to employ variety of molecular biological techniques to understand the biological processes intricately linked to oocyte, ovarian follicle development, fertilization and embryo development in general. Despite an abundance of knowledge concerning essential pathways which may have critical roles in regulation of fertility and necessary homeostasis, the repertoire of medications to treat female fertility problems remains limited to a few classes of drugs involved in the induction or suppression of folliculogenesis and ovulation; many of which are not specific in their drug actions and can give rise to complications during clinical application.

Studies on LIF proved that: 1) LIF gene mutations are significantly more frequent in infertile women compared to fertile controls; 2) LIF gene mutations are not restricted to primary or secondary infertility or to any specific infertility diagnosis; and 3) LIF gene mutations do not affect the outcome of infertility treatment in most patients but do in a subgroup of infertile women diagnosed with endometriosis or idiopathic infertility, In addition, the IVF outcome is statistically significantly lower than in control population of women with same diagnosis but no LIF gene mutation [6].

A fundamental aim of current research in infertility treatment is to develop new therapeutic approaches based on the knowledge of its etiopathogenesis. Further studies are needed to identify susceptibility gene(s) and the mechanism involved in endometriosis. DNA mutational analysis of these genes as well as the analysis of their functions will contribute to understanding the implantation failure in women with endometriosis and infertility in general.

Acknowledgment

Supported by the project CZ.1.05/2.1.00/03.0076 from European Regional Development Fund.

References

[1] Moragianni V. A., Penzias A. S. Cumulative live-birth rates after assisted reproductive technology. *Curr. Opin. Obstet. Gynecol.,* 2010 22, 189-192.

[2] Brown R., Harper J. The clinical benefit and safety of current and future assisted reproductive technology. *Reprod. Biomed. Online,* 2012, in press.

[3] Borini A., Lagalla C., Cattoli M., Sereni E., Scieajno R., Flamigni C., Coticchio G. Predictive factors for embryo implantation potential. *Reprod. Biomed. Online,* 2005, 10, 653-668.

[4] Corcoran D., Fair T. A., Lonergan P. Predicting embryo quality: mRNA expression and the preimplantation embryo. *Reprod. Biomed. Online,* 2005, 11:240-438.

[5] Kralickova M., Sima R., Vanecek T., Sima P., Rokyta Z., Ulcova-Gallova Z., Sucha R., Uher P., Hes O. Leukemia inhibitory factor gene mutations in the population of infertile women are not restricted to nulligravid patients. *Eur. J.Obstet. Gynecol. Reprod. Biol.,* 2006, 127, 231-235.

[6] Novotný Z., Křižan J., Šíma R., Šíma P., Uher P., Zech N., Hűttelová R., Baborová P., Ulčová-Gallová Z., Šubrt I., Ulmanová E., Houdek Z., Rokyta Z., Králíčková M. Leukemia inhibitory factor (lif) gene mutations in women diagnosed with unexplained infertility and endometriosis have negative impact on the IVF outcome. A pilot study. *Folia Biol.*, 2009, 55, 92-97.

[7] Simpson J. L. Molecular approach to common causes of female infertility. *Best Pract. Res Clin. Obstet. Gynaecol.*, 2002, 16, 685-702.

[8] Furnes B., Schimenti J. Fast forward to new genes in mammalian reproduction. *J.Physiol.*, 2007, 578, 25-32.

[9] Saso S., Ghaem-Maghami S., Chatterjee J., Brewig N., Ungar L., Smith J. R., el Priore G. Immunology of uterine transplantation: a review. *Reprod. Sci.*, 2012 19, 123-134.

[10] Matzuk M. M., Lamb D. J. The biology of infertility: Reseach advances and clinical challenges. *Nat. Med.*, 2008, 14, 1197-1213.

[11] Tabibzadeh S., Shea W., Lessey B. A., Broome J. From endometrial receptivity to infertility. *Semin. Reprod. Endocrinol.*, 1999, 17, 197-203.

[12] Makrigiannakis A., Minas V., Kalantaridou S. N., Nikas G., Chrousos G. P. Hormonal and cytokine regulation of early implantation. *Trends Endocrinol. Metab.*, 2006, 178-185.

[13] Makrigiannakis A., Minas V. Mechanisms of implantation. *Reprod. Biomed. Online*, 2007, 14, 75-82.

[14] Sharkey A. M., Smith S. K.The endometrium as a cause of implantation failure. *Best Pract. Res. Clin. Obstet. Gynaecol.*, 2003, 17, 289-307.

[15] Whibley C., Pharoah P. D., Hollstein M. p 53 polymorphisms: Cancer implications. *Nat. Rev. Cancer*, 2009, 9, 95-107.

[16] Marcel V., Hainaut P. p. 53 isoforms: a conspiracy to kidnap p53 tumor suppressor activity? *Cell. Mol. Life Sci.*, 2009, 66, 391-406.

[17] Stewart C. L. Reproduction: the unusual suspect. *Nature*, 2007, 450, 619.

[18] Feng Z., Zhang C., Kang H. J., Sun Y., Wang H., Naqvi A., Frank A. K., Rosenwaks Z., Murphy M. E., Levine A. J., Hu W. Regulation of female reproduction by p53 and its family members. *FASEB J.*, 2011, 25, 2245-2255.

[19] Kang H. J., Feng Z., Sun Y., Atwal G., Murphy M. E., Rebbeck T. R., Rosenwaks Z., Levine A. J., Hu W. Single-nucleotide polymorphisms in the p53 pathway regulate fertility in humans. *Proc. Natl. Acad. Sci. U. S. A.*, 2009, 106, 9761-9766.

[20] Hu W., Teresky A. K., Levine A. J. P53 regulates maternal reproduction through LIF. *Nature*, 2007, 450, 721-724.

[21] Hu W., Feng Z., Atwal G. S., Levine A. J. P53: A new player in reproduction. *Cell Cycle*, 2008, 7, 848-852.

[22] Nezhat F., Datta M. S., Hanson V., Pejovic T., Nezhat C. The relationship of endometriosis and ovarian malignancy: a review. *Fertil. Steril.*,2008, 90, 1559–1570.

[23] Tomida M., Yamamoto-Yamaguchi Y., Hozumi M. Purification of a factor inducing differentiation of mouse myeloid leukemic M1 cells from conditioned medium of mouse fibroblast L929 cells. *J. Biol. Chem.*,1984,*259,10978–10982.*

[24] *Stewart C. L., Kaspar P., Brunet L. J., Bhatt H., Gadi I., Kontgen F., Abbondanzo S. J. Blastocyst implantation depends on maternal expression of leukaemia inhibitory factor. Nature*, 1992, 359, 76-79.

[25] Sherwin J. R., Freeman T. C., Stephens R. J., Kimber S., Smith A. G., Chambers I., Smith S. K., Sharkey A. M. Identification of genes regulated by leukemia-inhibitory factor in the mouse uterus at the time of implantation. *Mol. Endocrinol.,* 2004, 18, 2185-2195.

[26] Hambartsoumian E., Taupin J. L., Moreau J. F., Frydman R., Chaouat G. *In-vivo* administration of progesterone inhibits the secretion of endometrial leukaemia inhibitory factor *in vitro*. *Mol. Hum. Reprod.,* 1998, 4, 1039-1044.

[27] Laird S. M., Tuckerman E. M., Li T. C. Cytokine expression in the endometrium of women with implantation failure and recurrent miscarriage. *Repr. Bio Med. Online,* 2006, 13, 12-23.

[28] Aghajanova L. Leukemia inhibitory factor and human embryo implantation. *Ann.N. Y. Acad. Sci.,* 2004, 1034, 176-183.

[29] Lass A., Weiser W., Munafo A., Loumaye E. Leukemia inhibitory factor in human reproduction. *Fertil. Steril.,* 2001, 76, 1091-1096.

[30] Giess R., Tanasescu I., Steck T., Sendtner M. Leukaemia inhibitory factor gene mutations in infertile women. *Mol Hum Reprod.,* 1999 5, 581-586.

[31] Steck T., Giess R., Suetterlin M. W., Bolland M., Wiest S., Poehls U. G., Dietl J. Leukaemia inhibitory factor (LIF) gene mutations in women with unexplained infertility and recurrent failure of implantation after IVF and embryo transfer. *Eur. J.Obstet. Gynecol. Reprod. Biol.,* 2004, 112, 69-73.

[32] von Rango U., Alfer J., Kertschanska S., Kemp B., Muller-Newen G., Heinrich P. C. Beier H. M., Classen-Linke I. Interleukin-11 expression: its significance in eutopic and ectopic human implantation. *Mol. Hum. Reprod.,* 2004, 10, 783-792.

[33] Karpovich N., Klemmt P., Hwang J. H., McVeigh J. E., Heath J. K., Barlow D. H., Mardon H. J. The production of interleukin-11 and decidualization are compromised in endometrial stromal cells derived from patients with infertility. *J. Clin. Endocrinol. Metab.,* 2005, 90, 1607-1612.

[34] Dimitriadis E., Sharkey A. M., Tan Y. L., Salamnosen L. A., Sherwin J. R. A. Immunolocalisation of phosphorylated STAT3, interleukin 11 and leukaemia inhibitory factor in endometrium of women with unexplained infertility during the implantation window. Reprod. Biol. Endocrinol., 2007, 5, 44.

[35] Dimitriadis E., Stoikos C., Stafford-Bell M., Clark I., Paiva P., Kovacs G., Salamonsen L. A. Interleukin-11, IL-11 receptor alpha and leukemia inhibitory factor are dysregulated in endometrium of infertile women with endometriosis during the implantation window. *J. Reprod. Immunol.,* 2006, 69, 53-64.

[36] Wang Q., Sun Q. Y. Evaluation of oocyte quality: morphological, cellular and molecular predictors. *Reprod. Fertil. Dev.,* 2007, 19, 1–12.

[37] Ledee N., Lombroso R., Lombardelli L., Selva J., Dubanchet S., Chaouat G, Frankenne F, Foidart J. M., Romagnani S., Ville Y., Piccinni M. P. Cytokines and chemokines in follicular fluids and potential of the corresponding embryo: the role of granulocyte colony-stimulating factor. *Human Reprod.,* 2008, 23, 2001-2009.

[38] Salmassi A., Acil Y., Schmutzler A. G., Koch K., Jonat W., Mettler L. Differential interleukin-6 messenger ribonucleic acid expression and its distribution pattern in eutopic and ectopic endometrium. *Fertil. Steril.,* 2008, 89, 1578-1584.

[39] Asimakopoulos B., Koster F., Felberbaum R., Tripsiannis G., Caglar G. S., Nikolettos N., Al-Hasani S., Diedrich K. Intrafollicular and circulating concentrations of leptin do not predict the outcome in IVF-ICSI cycles. *Reprod. Sci.,* 2009, 16, 113-119.

[40] Asimakopoulos B., Abu-Hassan D., Metzen E., Al-Hasani S., Diedrich K., Nikolettos N. The level of steroid hormones and cytokines in individual follicles are not associated with the fertilization outcome after intracytoplasmic sperm injection. *Fertil. Steril.,* 2008, 90, 60-64.

[41] Asimakopoulos B., Nikolettos N., Papachristou D. N., Simopoulou M., Al-Hasani S., Diedrich K. Follicular fluid levels of vascular endothelial growth factor and leptin are associated with pregnancy outcome of normal women participating in intracytoplasmic sperm injection cycles. *Physiol. Res.*, 2005, 54, 263-270.

[42] Wunder D. M., Guibourdenche J., Birkhauser M. H., Bersinger N. A. Anti-Mullerian hormone and inhibin B as predictors of pregnancy after treatment by *in vitro* fertilization/intracytoplasmic sperm injection. *Fertil. Steril.*, 2008, 90, 2203–2210.

[43] Anifandis G., Koutselini E., Stefanidis I., Liakopoulos V., Leivaditis C., Mantzavinos T., Vamvakopoulos N. Serum and follicular fluid leptin levels are correlated with human embryo quality. *Reproduction,* 2005, 130, 917-921.

[44] Salmassi A., Schmutzler A. G., Schaefer S., Koch K., Hedderich J., Jonat W., Mettler L. Is granulocyte colony-stimulating factor level predictive for human IVF outcome? *Hum. Reprod.,* 2005, 20, :2434-2440.

[45] Lewicka S., von Hagens C., Hettinger U., Grunwald K., Vecsei P., Runnebaum B., Rabe T. Cortisol and cortisone in human follicular fluid and serum and the outcome of IVF treatment. *Hum.Reprod.,* 2003, 18, 1613–1617.

[46] Fried G., Remaeus K., Harlin J., Krog E., Csemiczky G., Aanesen A., Tally M. Inhibin B predicts oocyte number and the ratio IGF-I/IGFBP-1 may indicate oocyte quality duting ovarian hyperstimulation for *in vitro* fertilization. *J. Assist. Reprod. Genet.,* 2003, 20, 167-176.

[47] Hsieh Y. Y., Chang C. C., Tsai H. D., Lin C. S. Leukemia inhibitory factor in follicular fluid is not related to the number and quality of embryos as well as implantation and pregnancy rates. *Biochem. Genet.*, 2005, 43, 501-506.

[48] Ledee-Bataille N., Lapree-Delage G., Taupin J. L., Dubanchet S., Taieb J., Moreau J. F., Chaouat G. Follicular fluid concentration of leukemia inhibitory factor is decreased among women with polycystic ovaian syndrome during assisted reproduction cycles. *Human Reprod.,* 2001, 16, 2073-2078.

[49] Ozornek M. H., Bielfeld P., Krussel J. S., Hirschenhain J., Jeyendran R. S., Koldovsky U. Epidermal growth factor and leukemia inhibitory factor levels in follicular fluid. Association with *in vitro* fertilization outcome. *J. Reprod. Med.,* 1999, 44, 367-369.

[50] MacLeod, J. The role of oxygen in the metabolism and motility of human spermatozoa. *Am. J. Physiol.,* 1943, 138, 512-518.

[51] Halliwell B., Gutteridge J. M. C. *Free radicals in biology and medicine*, 2nd Edn. Oxford, OxfordUniversity Press, 1989.

[52] Knapen M. F., Zusterzeel P. L., Peters W. H., Steegers E. A. Glutathione and glutathione-related enzymes in reproduction. A review. *Eur. J. Obstet. Gynecol. Reprod. Biol.,* 1999, 82, 171–184.

[53] Ho Y. S., Gargano M., Cao J., Bronson R. T., Heimler I., Hutz R. J. Reduced fertility in female mice lacking copper-zinc superoxide dismutase. *J. Biol. Chem.,* 1998, 273, 7765-7769.

[54] Matzuk M. M., Dionne L., Guo Q., Kumar T. R., Lebovitz R. M. Ovarian function in superoxide dismutase 1 and 2 knockout mice. *Endocrinology,* 1998, 139, 4008-4011.

[55] Angelucci S., Ciavardelli D., di Giuseppe F., Eleuterio E., Sulpizio M., Tiboni G. M., Giampietro F., Palumbo P., di Illio C. Proteome analysis of human follicular fluid. *Biochim. Biohys. Acta,* 2006, 1764, 1775-1785.

[56] Tatemoto H., Sakurai N., Muto N. Protection of porcine oocytes against apoptotic cell death caused by oxidative stress during *in vitro* maturation: role of cumulus cells. *Biol. Reprod.,* 2000, 63, 805–810.

[57] Appasamy M., Jauniaux E., Serhal P., Al-Qahtani A., Groome N. P., Muttukrishna S. Evaluation of the relationship between follicular fluid oxidative stress, ovarian hormones, and response to gonadotropin stimulation. *Fertil. Steril.,* 2008, 89, 912-921.

[58] Das S., Chattopadhyay R., Ghosh S., Ghosh S., Goswami S. K., Chakravarty B. N., Chaudhury K. Reactive oxygen species level in follicular fluid – embryo wuality marker in IVF? *Human Reprod.,* 2006, 21:2403-2407.

[59] Pasqualotto E. B., Lara L. V., Salvador M., Sobreiro B. P., Borges E., Pasqualotto F. F. The role of enzymatic antioxidants detected in the follicular fluid and semen of infertile couples undergoing assisted reproduction. *Hum. Fertil.,* 2009, 12, 166–171.

[60] Tamura H., Takasaki A., Miwa I., Taniguchi K., Maekawa R., Asada H., Taketani T., Matsuoka A., Yamagata Y., Shimurama K., Morioka H., Ishikawa H., Reiter R. J., Sugino N. Oxidative stress impairs oocyte quality and melatonin protects oocytes from free radical damage and improves fertilization rate. *J. Pineal Res.,* 2008, 44, 280-287.

[61] Basini G., Simona B., Santini S. E., Grasselli F. Reactive oxygen species and anti-oxidant defences in swine follicular fluids. *Reprod. Fertil. Dev.,* 2008, 20, 269–274.

[62] Baka S., Malamitsi-Puchner A. Novel follicular fluid factors influencing oocyte developmental potential in IVF: a review. *Reprod. Biomed. Online.* 2006, 12, 500-506.

[63] Oral O., Kutlu T., Aksoy E., Ficicioglu C., Uslu H., Tugrul S. The effects of oxidative stress on outcomes of assisted reproductive techniques. *J. Assist. Reprod. Genet.,* 2006, 23, 81-85.

[64] Seino T., Saito H., Kaneko T., Takahashi T., Kawachiya S., Kurachi H. Eight-hydroxy-2'-deoxyguanosine in granulosa cells is correlated with the quality of oocytes and embryos in an *in vitro* fertilization-embryo transfer program. *Fertil. Steril.,* 2002, 77, 1184–1190.

[65] Paszkowski T., Traub A. I., Robinson S. Y., McMaster D. Selenium dependent glutathione peroxidase activity in human follicular fluid. *Clin. Chim. Acta,* 1995, 236, 173–180.

[66] Paszkowski T., Clarke R. N. Antioxidant capacity of preimplantation embryo culture medium declines following the incubation of poor quality embryos. *Hum. Reprod.,* 1996, 11, 2493–2495.

[67] Wiener-Megnazi Z., Vardi L., Lissak A., Schnizer S., Reznick A. Z., Ishai D., Lahav-Baratz S., Shilog H., Koifman M., Dirnfeld M. Oxidative stress indices in follicular fluid as measured by the thermochemiluminiscence assay correlate with outcome parameters in *in vitro* fertilization. *Fertil. Steril.,* 2004, 82 (Suppl. 3), 1171-1176.

[68] Broekmans F. J., Kwee J., Hendriks D. J., Mol B. W., Lambalk C. B. A systematic review of tests predicting ovarian reserve and IVF outcome. *Human Reprod. Update,* 2006, 12, 685-718.

[69] Paszkowski T., Clarke R. N., Hornstein M. D. Smokind induces oxidative stress inside the Graafian follicle. *Human Reprod.,* 2002, 17, 921-925.

[70] Tiboni G. M., Bucciarelli T., Giampietro F., Sulpizio M., Di Ilio C. Influence of cigarette smoking on vitamin E, vitamin A, beta-carotene and lycopene concentrations in human preovulatory follicular fluid. *Int. J. Immunopathol. Pharmacol.,* 2004, 17, 389–393.

[71] Agca C., Ries J. E., Kolath S. J., Kim J. H., Forrester L. J., Antoniou E., Whitworth K. M., Mathialagan N., Springer G. K., Prather R. S., Lucy M. C. Luteinization of porcine preovulatory follicles lead to systematic changes in follicular gene expression. *Reproduction,* 2006, 132, 133-145.

[72] Gupta S., Choi A., Yu H. Y., Czerniak S. M., Holick E. A., Paolella L. J., Agarwal A., Combelles C. M. Fluctuation in total antioxidant capacity, catalase activity and hydrogen peroxide levels of follicular fluid during bovine folliculogenesis. *Reprod. Fertil. Dev.,* 2011, 23, 673-680.

[73] Yang H. W., Hwang K. J., Kwon H. C., Kim H. S., Choi K. W., Oh K. S. Detection of reactive oxygen speciees (ROS) and apoptosis in human fragmented embryos. *Human Reprod.,* 1998, 13, 998-1002.

[74] Bischoff F. Z., Simpson J. L. Heritability and molecular genetic studies of endometriosis. *Hum. Reprod. Update,* 2000, 6, 37-44.

[75] Mahutte N. G., Arici A. New advances in the understanding of endometriosis related infertility. *J. Reprod. Immunol.,* 2002, 55, 73-83.

[76] Senapati S., Barnhart K. Managing endometriosis-associated infertility. *Clin. Obstet. Gynecol.,* 2011, 54, 720-726.

[77] Seli E., Arici A. Endometriosis: interaction of immune and endocrine systems. *Semin. Reprod. Med.,* 2003, 21, 135-144.

[78] Wu M. Y., Ho H. N. The role of cytokines in endometriosis. *Am. J. Reprod. Immunol.,* 2003, 49, 285-296.

[79] Matarese G., de Placido G., Nikas Y., Alviggi C. Pathogenesis of endometriosis: natural immunity dysfunction or autoimmune disease? *Trends Mol. Med.,* 2003, 9, 223-228.

[80] Ulukus M., Arici A. Immunology of endometriosis. *Minerva Gynecol.,* 2005, 57, 237-248.

[81] Sikora J., Mielczarek-Palacz A., Kondera-Anasz Z. Role of natural killer cell activity in the pathogenesis of endometriosis. *Curr. Med. Chem.,* 2011, 18, 200-208.

[82] Illera M. J., Juan L., Stewart C. L., Cullinan E., Ruman J., Lessey B. A. Effect of peritoneal fluid from women with endometriosis on implantation in the mouse model. *Fertil. Steril.,* 2000, 74, 41-48.

[83] Mikolajczyk M., Wirstlein P., Skrzypczak J. Leukaemia inhibitory factor and interleukin 11 levels in uterine flushings of infertile patients with endometriosis. *Hum. Reprod.,* 2006, 21, 3054-3058.

[84] Johnson P. M., Christmas S. E., Vince G. S. Immunological aspects of implantation and implantation failure. *Hum. Reprod.,* 1999, Suppl. 2, 26-36.

[85] Flynn L., Byrne B., Carton J., Kelehan P., O'Herlihy C., O'Farrelly C. Menstrual cycle dependent fluctuations in NK and T-lymphocyte subsets from non-pregnant human endometrium. *Am. J. Reprod. Immunol.,* 2000, 43, 209-217.

[86] Croy B. A., Esadeg S., Chantakru S., van den Heuvel M., Paffaro V. A., He H., Black G. P., Ashkar A. A., Kiso Y., Zhang J. Update on pathways regulating the activation of uterine natural killer cells, their interactions with decidual spiral arteries and homing of their precursors to the uterus. *J. Reprod. Immunol.,* 2003, 59, 175-191.

[87] Giudice L. C., Telles T. L., Lobo S., Kao L. *The molecular basis for implantation failure in endometriosis: on the road to discovery.*

[88] Surrey E. S., Schoolcraft W. B. *Ann. N. Y. Acad. Sci.,* 2002, 955, 252-264.Management of endometriosis-associated infertility. *Obstet. Gynecol. Clin. North Am.,* 2003, 30, 193-208.

[89] Zhang C., Maeda N., Izumiya C., Yamamoto Y., Kusume T., Oguri H., Yamashita C., Nishimori Y., Hayashi K., Luo J., Fukaya T. Killer immunoglobulin-like receptor and human leukocyte antigen expression as immunodiagnostic parameters for pelvic endometriosis. *Am. J. Reprod. Immunol.,* 2006, 55, 106-114.

[90] Matsuoka S., Maeda N., Izumiya C., Yamashita C., Nishimori Y, Fukaya T. Expression of inhibitory-motif killer immunoglobulin-like receptor, KIR2DL1, is increased in natural killer cells from women with pelvic endometriosis. *Am. J. Reprod. Immunol.,* 2005, 53, 249-254.

[91] Maeda N., Izumiya C., Oguri H., Kusume T., Yamamoto Y., Fukaya T. Aberrant expression of intercellular adhesion molecule-1 and killer inhibitory receptors induces immune tolerance in women with pelvic endometriosis. *Fertil. Steril.,* 2002, 77, 679-683.

[92] Maeda N., Izumiya C., Taniguchi K., Matsushima S., Fukaya T. Role of NK cells and HLA-G in endometriosis. *Front. Biosci.,* 2012, 4, 1568-1581.

[93] Schofield G., Kimber S. J. Leukocyte subpopulations in the uteri of leukemia inhibitory factor knockout mice during early pregnancy. *Biol. Reprod.,* 2005, 72, 872-878.

[94] Fraccaroli L., Grasso E., Zeitler E., Lombardi E., Gogorza S., Etchepareborda J. J., Nagle C., Cortelezzi M., Pérez Leirós C., Ramhorst R. Modulation of maternal LIF producers T cells by trophoblast and paternal antigens. *Am. J. Reprod. Immunol.,* 2011, 65, 133-145.

[95] Dimitriadis E., Menkhorst E., Salamonsen L. A., Paiva P. Review: LIF and IL-11 in trophoblast-ndometrial interactions during the establishment of pregnancy. *Placenta,* 2010, 31, S99-S104.

[96] Sharkey A. M., King A., Clark D. E., Burrows T. D., Jokhi P. P., Charnock-Jones D. S., Loke Y. W., Smith S. K.: Localization of leukemia inhibitory factor and its receptor in human placenta throughout pregnancy. *Biol. Reprod.,* 1999, 60, 355-364.

[97] Saito S., Nishikawa K., Morii T., Enomoto M., Narita N., Motoyoshi K., Ichijo M. Cytokine production by CD16-CD56bright natural killer cells in the human early pregnancy decidua. *Int. Immunol.,* 1993, 5, 559-563.

[98] Jokhi P. P., King A., Sharkey A. M., Smith S. K., Loke Y. W.: Screening for cytokine messenger ribonucleic acids in purified human decidual lymphocyte populations by the reverse-transcriptase polymerase chain reaction. *J. Immunol.,* 1994, 153, 4427-4435.

[99] Fedele L., Berlanda N. Emerging drugs for endometriosis. *Expert Opin. Emerg. Drugs,* 2004, 9,167-177.

[100] Barrier B. F., Kendall B. S., Ryan C. E., Sharpe-Timms K. L. HLA-G is expressed by the glandular epithelium of peritoneal endometriosis but not in eutopic endometrium. *Hum. Reprod.,* 2006, 21, 864-869.

[101] Giudice L. C., Kao L. C. Endometriosis. *Lancet,* 2004, 364, 1789-1799.

In: Infertility
Editors: R. Nascimento and H. V. Boas
ISBN: 978-1-62257-909-9

Chapter 4

The Potential Effect of Clinician-Induced (Iatrogenic) Damage Incurred During Fertility Treatment Upon Gamete Competence and Embryonic Viability

Celine Jones, Hani Bagheri, Junaid Kashir, Laura McLaren, Suseela Yelumalai and Kevin Coward*
[1]Nuffield Department of Obstetrics and Gynaecology, Women's Centre, John Radcliffe Hospital, Headington, Oxford, UK

Abstract

Infertility affects an estimated 9% of couples worldwide. While advances in assisted reproductive technology (ART) have revolutionised the treatment of infertility, success rates are highly variable. Pregnancy and delivery rates for common techniques such as *in vitro* fertilisation (IVF) and intracytoplasmic sperm injection (ICSI) rarely exceed 30% and 23% respectively. An increasing body of evidence strongly suggests that routine ART techniques may inadvertently induce detrimental effects upon gametes and embryos, compromising either gamete fertility or embryonic viability. Consequently, it is critical that ART protocols are constantly refined or replaced in line with scientific advances, such that clinics can provide patients with an optimised chance of successful conception. Here, we discuss a number of ways in which ART protocols are known to induce detrimental effect upon critical biomarkers of gamete and embryo health, and identify future areas for investigative research. As the number of couples seeking fertility treatment worldwide increases, the efficacy of ART is more important than ever. By informing the research community of the potential ways in which ART may compromise gamete and embryo viability, it is the intention of this commentary to inspire concerted research effort such that ART protocols can be refined or replaced as necessary.

*E-mail:kevin.coward@obs-gyn.ox.ac.uk

Keywords: Assisted reproductive technology (ART), iatrogenic damage, sperm, oocytes, embryos

Introduction

According to the human fertilisation and embryology association (HFEA, 2010), infertility affects one in seven couples, amounting to ~70 million couples worldwide (Kashir *et al.*, 2010; Ledger *et al.*, 2009). Natural conception may fail for a variety of reasons, and can be attributed to male and/or female factors, unexplained infertility, and a host of other parameters (HFEA 2010). In females, infertility can arise by mechanical (endometriosis, or uterine lining defects), ovulary (anovulation), or cervical (polyps and cysts) factors (Healy *et al.*, 1994). In males, deficiencies may arise from a total lack of sperm in semen (azoospermia), a low concentration of sperm (oligozoospermia), poor sperm motility (asthenozoospermia), or abnormal sperm morphology (teratozoospermia). Such factors may be caused by a variety of underlying problems, including anomalous enlargement of veins in the scrotum (varicocele) resulting in compromised blood drainage in the testicles, testicular insufficiency conditions where one or both testes from the scrotum are absent (cryptorchidism), or idiopathic (unknown) factors (Kashir *et al.*, 2010). Since the birth of Louise Brown in 1978, the first *in vitro* fertilisation (IVF) baby, many other techniques have been developed and are regularly used in assisted reproductive technology (ART) laboratories. One such technique is intracytoplasmic sperm injection (ICSI), in which a single sperm is microinjected directly into the cytoplasm of the oocyte. However, despite the introduction of such revolutionary techniques, ART success rates still remain around the 30% level observed by Edwards over 30 years ago (Edwards *et al.*,1984; Inge *et al.*, 2005; Kashir *et al.*, 2011). It is thus essential that success rates are further improved such that ART can provide the best care for the increasing population of couples afflicted by infertility (Kashir *et al.*, 2011). During ART procedures, gametes and embryos are removed from their natural environment and placed into an artificial one, raising the distinct possibility that external factors may induce clinician-induced (iatrogenic) damage, which may compromise their quality and viability. Indeed, such interventions may themselves represent the underlying causative factors behind the relatively low success rates observed during ART, despite significant improvements in laboratory settings, equipment, and clinical expertise. One highly plausible reason underlying poor success may be detrimental changes within the *in vitro* culture environment. However, such environmental factors are likely to be diverse in nature and thus challenging to isolate and eliminate. Alongside environmental factors surrounding embryo culture, changes to laboratory procedures and equipment utilisation may exert some degree of influence upon ART outcomes. While a significant body of research has investigated the potential effects of environmental factors upon ART success, laboratory protocols remain relatively unchanged (Rienzi *et al.*, 2011).

Embryo Culture

Up to ~75% of human embryos produced *in vitro* may undergo embryo fragmentation (a chaotic division of embryonic cells) (Alikani *et al.*, 2007) and more than 15% of fragmentation cases have been associated with an increased risk of embryonic developmental failure (Alikani *et al.*, 1999). However, the exact causes underlying embryo fragmentation are not known, and it is unclear whether fragmentation arises inadvertently due to culture conditions and follicular stimulation in ART, or whether it is a normal characteristic of human embryo development (Keefe and Liu, 2008) (Figure 1). Excessive changes in the levels of free radicals, temperature, and pH, have all been proposed to contribute towards embryo fragmentation (Keefe and Liu, 2008). A further possible causative factor may include mineral oil, which is commonly used during embryo culture. Elevated levels of oil hyper-oxides are believed to be triggered in culture media by exposure to oxygen, sunlight, UV-light, or inadequate storage. Such effects are known to be enhanced with increased exposure. Therefore, careful evaluation of mineral oils, and their storage between cycles of use, is highly warranted for ART (Otsuki *et al.*, 2007). Furthermore, Otsuki *et al.* (2009) reported that the presence of albumin in culture media facilitates the uptake of oil peroxidation-derived free-radicals into the zona-pellucida, a mechanism related to the structural properties of albumin, which can consequently cause harm to cultured embryos and oocytes. Consequently, the use of additional protein supplements in culture media is not recommended for ART (Otsuki *et al.*, 2009). Mineral oil, however, is still used for embryo culture since no viable alternative has been identified, although a recent study has shown that mineral oil-induced embryo-toxicity can be significantly reduced by washing the oil with synthetic human tubal fluid (Morbeck *et al.*, 2010). Further studies are required to assess the outcome of such procedures upon embryo health (Morbeck *et al.*, 2010) and to determine if further improvements can be expected from further changes in the use or treatment of mineral oil. The 'microdrop' method, deployed extensively for ICSI and insemination procedures, is highly advantageous as it allows culture medium to remain at constant levels of pH and osmolarity. However, such methodology can also exert detrimental effect upon embryos by inducing toxic contamination of the medium (Otsuki *et al.*, 2007).

While considering the potential threat imposed by environmental factors upon embryo culture in ART, it is important to develop an understanding of the physical conditions embryos face *in vivo*. For example, embryos are exposed to cilial movement and muscle contraction *in vivo*, and thus the creation of a dynamic culture which mimics such an environment more closely while preventing the creation of isolated areas of depleted nutrients, or areas of increased toxin content, may contribute towards improved success (Smith *et al.*, 2012). Tilting and shaking of embryos seems to exert only minimal effect upon viability, but vibrational agitation may be associated with increased pregnancy rates (Smith *et al.*, 2012). The use of microfluidic dynamic culture systems, endometrial cell line co-cultures (Smith *et al.*, 2012), and automated micro-channel systems, which could be deployed during embryo development prior to implantation and thus reducing the need for manual handling, is a growing area of investigation (Thompson, 2007; Rienzi *et al.*, 2011). However, even simple micro-culture techniques are not in widespread use as cost considerations favour the use of more established equipment (Thompson, 2007; Rienzi *et al.*, 2011).

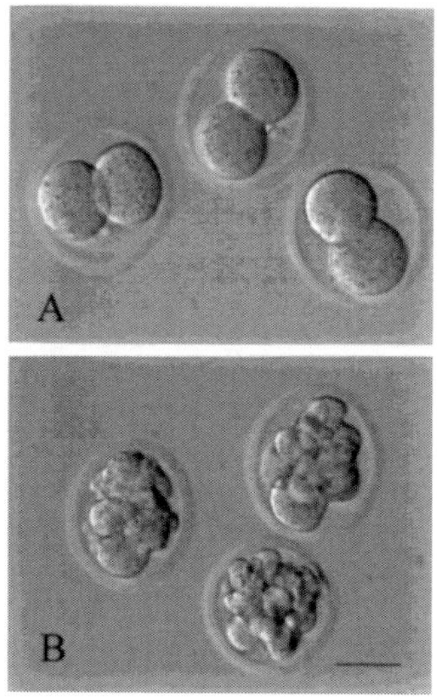

Figure 1. Representative images showing non-fragmented (A), and fragmented (B), mouse embryos at the two-cell stage. Scale bar represents 50μm. Figure reproduced from Alikani *et al.* (2005) with permission.

The use of higher embryo:culture ratios has been linked to improved success, possibly due to the 'co-operative interaction' of growth factors released in a paracrine or autocrine fashion (Paria *et al.*, 1990; Lane *et al.*, 1992; Gardner *et al.*, 1994; Smith *et al.*, 2012), or the dilution of toxic factors (Bavister *et al.*,1995; Vajta *et al.*, 2010). Novel methodology utilises micro-drops (10 to 50μl in volume) to take advantage of potentially beneficial embryo-secreted factors. Although some reports have suggested this may result in increased abnormality (Vajta *et al.*, 2010), this technique more than doubled the pregnancy rate for bovine embryos (Vajta *et al.*, 2000 ; Smith *et al.*, 2012). However, laboratories have been slow to implement such techniques owing to the practice of culturing embryos individually for identification purposes (Rienzi *et al.*, 2011).

At present, laboratories are responsible for deciding which culture techniques they prefer to adopt, despite evidence that environmental factors affect not only ART success rates, but also the size and weight of the developing fetus, which themselves may be a strong indicator of future health. A consensus is desperately needed, as alongside possible physical damage to cells affecting implantation success rates, environmental factors may also cause genetic/epigenetic defects which could affect future health of the child and, by inheritance, future generations. Furthermore, unified codes of practice would allow success rates from individual laboratories to be utilised within a parameterised database, which would greatly aid the identification of beneficial procedures and techniques.

Sperm Processing in ART

ART techniques are readily deployed to separate sperm from the seminal plasma of sub-fertile males with low sperm counts, or to gather the healthiest sperm for downstream treatment (Twigg *et al.*, 1998). The most common techniques utilised include swim-up, and density-gradient washing (DGW) or centrifugation (DGC). Swim-up and DGW techniques are advantageous as sperm motility is retained for up to 24 hours following cryopreservation (Sharma *et al.*, 1996). However, all three methods increase the production of reactive oxygen species (ROS) within sperm (Shekarriz *et al.*, 1995; Zini *et al.*, 1999; 2000; Li *et al.*, 2011), which correlate to chromatin cross-linking and base pair changes within the sperm nucleus (Twigg *et al.*, 1998). DNA damage caused by sperm gathering techniques (Aitken *et al.*, 1994; 1995) is dependent upon initial sperm quality (Zini *et al.*, 2000), which in the case of infertile men, is generally low. Indeed, DNA damage may be exacerbated in cases of leukocytospermia (presence of high leukocytes counts in seminal fluid) or when sperm are separated from protective antioxidants in the plasma (Aitken *et al.*, 1995; Twigg *et al.*, 1998).

Density-Gradient Centrifugation (DGC) and Swim-up (SUP) Protocols

Sperm washing is a routinely used procedure in infertility treatment. Two of the most commonly used sperm washing techniques are swim-up (SUP) and density-gradient centrifugation (DGC), both of which are carried out prior to ART procedures such as IVF or ICSI (Boomsma *et al.*, 2007). Both techniques are performed to separate good-quality from sub-optimal sperm by isolation from seminal plasma (and ejaculate debris) to avoid over-exposure and toxic effects, hence increasing the chance of successful fertilisation (Allamaneni *et al.*, 2005). SUP methodology isolates motile sperm by facilitating the "swim-up" of highly motile sperm into culture medium leaving slow and non-motile sperm behind (Enciso *et al.*, 2011). DGC separates high-quality sperm (in terms of morphology and motility) from those that are sub-optimal, based upon relative buoyant density (Tavalaee *et al.*, 2012). However, both techniques may increase sperm DNA damage (Tavalaee *et al.*, 2012) via the removal of sperm from the seminal plasma which contains protective enzymes and antioxidants (such as superoxide dismutase, catalyse, and ascorbate). As a consequence, reactive oxygen species (ROS) produced by damaged sperm may transfer or elevate oxidative stress and DNA damage to adjacent undamaged sperm (Hughes *et al.*, 1998).

Considering that semen from infertile men generally exhibit higher ROS levels with respect to fertile men, DGC may exacerbate the reduced quality of viable sperm produced by infertile males (Younglai *et al.*, 2001). Moreover, sperm washing protocols may induce a two-fold increase in DNA damage in normal sperm samples from fertile men (Tavalaee *et al.*, 2012). Since sperm are transcriptionally inactive and deficient of functional enzymatic repair systems, such methods may confer some degree of risk for permanent damage (Drost and Lee, 1995). Damage to sperm caused by these techniques can, however, be reduced by reducing centrifugation time or by the addition of antioxidants to the sperm culture medium (Gadea *et al.*, 2011). Currently, there is no firm evidence to recommend any specific preparation method for sperm. Large high-quality randomised controlled trials are required to compare the effects of these techniques upon clinical outcomes (Boomsma *et al.*, 2007; Enciso *et al.*, 2011).

Cryopreservation and Fertility Preservation

Cryopreservation is the act of freezing cells or tissues to sub-zero temperatures (commonly to -196 ˚C using liquid nitrogen) to preserve and store biological specimens for extended time periods (Jain and Paulson, 2006). The extremely low temperatures involved in cryopreservation prevent any biological activity, such as cell death, and thus enable gametes and blastocysts to be preserved until a much later date. This technique is especially relevant for cancer patients about to begin chemo- or radio-therapy treatments which irreversibly damage the production of viable gametes (Pacey, 2010). Cryopreservation, however, is a harsh and damaging procedure which can cause extensive cellular damage to a living biological tissue or cell. To minimise physical damage resulting from the formation of ice crystals during freeze-thaw procedures, cryoprotectant agents such as glycerol or propylene glycol are normally added to the material being preserved (Jain and Paulson, 2006). Some cryoprotectant agents are potentially dangerous chemicals which may increase the risk of chemical cytotoxicity to the preserved cells (Huang *et al.*, 2006). Consequently, it is crucial to select the correct combination of cryoprotectants based on species type, the length of exposure, and the stage of embryonic development (Cean *et al.*, 2011).

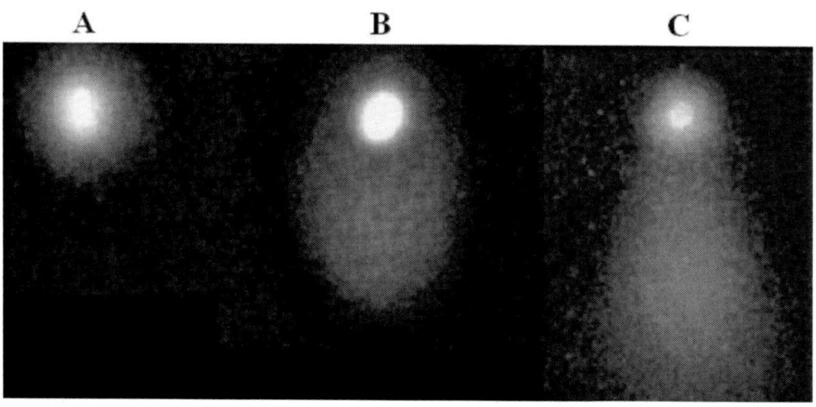

Figure 2. Representative micrographs of human sperm following an electrophoresis comet assay for DNA fragmentation. The majority of DNA from normal sperm migrates as a single cohesive mass, while in sperm with DNA fragmentation, a comet-like structure is created with the fragmented DNA forming the "tail". The further the migration, the more profound the damage produced. (A) Undamaged DNA, (B) intermediate DNA damage, and (C) extensive DNA damage in human sperm. Figure reproduced from Enciso *et al.* (2009) with permission.

Cryopreservation may also induce oxidative stress in sperm by increasing the number of ROS and reducing the concentration of antioxidants, such as glutathione (Gadea *et al.*, 2011). Changes in the concentration of oxidants/antioxidants results in damage to cellular lipids and proteins (Gadea *et al.*, 2011), increased incidence of DNA fragmentation, which reduces sperm viability and function (Zribi *et al.*, 2010), and can reduce ART success by causing poor rates of conception, poor embryonic development, childhood mortality and increased risk of miscarriage (Merlob *et al.*, 2005; Farr *et al.*, 2007; Collins *et al.*, 2008; Aitken *et al.*, 2009) (Figure 2). While some studies report that cryopreservation has no effect upon chromosomes and the ability of sperm to produce viable offspring (Kusakabe *et al.*, 2001), others suggest that DNA fragmentation measurements are under-estimated due to skewing of the TUNEL assay by DNA compaction and cell vitality (Mitchell *et al.*, 2011).

Cryopreservation techniques are being constantly developed in order to reduce potential risk to gametes and embryos. Cryoprotectants can replace water in cells during freezing (Kim *et al.*, 2011), and vitrification has been utilised to replace slow-freezing technologies (Herrero *et al.*, 2011), allowing higher cryoprotectant concentrations within cells and faster freezing to preserve cells in a 'glassy' state, which avoids the formation of damaging ice crystals (Herrero *et al.*, 2011; Larman *et al.*, 2007). Simplified or adapted vitrification protocols have reported even better survival and fertilisation rates compared to original protocols and there is thus significant hope for considerable further improvements in the near future (Lane *et al.*, 2001; Kim *et al.*, 2006; Lee *et al.*, 2007; Kim *et al.*, 2011).

The Effects of Freeze-Thawing upon Sperm

Several independent studies have examined the effects of freeze-thawing on sperm morphology, motility, viability, and ultrastructure (Hammadeh *et al.*, 1999; Ozkavukcu *et al.*, 2008; Zribi *et al.*, 2010). Generally, cryopreservation of sperm is associated with detrimental effects upon motility, morphology (plasmolemma, tails, and acrosomes), DNA integrity, and viability (Zribi *et al.*, 2010). Furthermore, Borges *et al.* (2007) showed that fertilisation rates following ICSI were higher using fresh sperm (73.8%) compared with frozen sperm (68.7%). Sperm with reduced motility (asthenozoospermic) and low sperm count with reduced motility (oligoasthenozoospermic) were shown to be more severely affected by cryopreservation, resulting in a lower fertilisation rate for frozen-thawed samples when compared with fresh samples (Borges *et al.*, 2007).

Of all the organelles that are sensitive to cryo-injury, the acrosome appears to be the most sensitive (Ozkavukcu *et al.*, 2008). The acrosome is an essential component of the sperm which facilitates penetration of the sperm into the oocyte by releasing digestive enzymes (e.g. acrosin) which break-up the oocyte membrane, leading to fertilisation. Thus, the destruction of the acrosome or sub-acrosomal components can lead to infertile sperm incapable of penetrating the oocyte (Kashir *et al.*, 2011). More recent studies by Gosálvez *et al.* (2011) and Johnston *et al.* (2012) have reported the presence of similar detrimental effects arising from cryopreservation upon sperm integrity and the dynamics of DNA fragmentation. Furthermore, Kashir *et al.* (2011) reported that the concentration of the putative sperm-specific oocyte activation factor, phospholipase C zeta (PLCζ), was significantly reduced (by 20-56%) following cryopreservation in human sperm. PLCζ is a protein localised in acrosomal, equatorial, and post-acrosomal regions of the sperm (Grasa *et al.*, 2008) and generates a prolonged series of intra-cellular calcium (Ca^{2+}) oscillations which leads to meiotic continuation and the beginning of embryogenesis (Swann *et al.*, 2006; Kashir *et al.*, 2011).

Gadea *et al.* (2011) also showed that the concentration of glutathione protein (GSH; an essential antioxidant component of semen) in human semen decreased considerably (by 64%) following cryopreservation. This reduction in GSH was correlated with a significant decline (by 68%) in sperm progressive motility. The effect of GSH on sperm motility was tested by adding GSH to the freezing extender (media) used to cryopreserve sperm. Such experiments resulted in improvements in total progressive motility, reduced levels of sperm ROS, and increased concentrations of sulfhydryl groups on membrane proteins, and hence generally increased sperm viability. Martinez-Soto (2011) indicated that cryopreserved sperm viability was significantly improved (~5%) following the deployment of a new freezing technique in which sperm were first centrifuged to form a pellet, immersed in thawing medium, and then thawed at 37 °C for 20 minutes. Clearly, such novel techniques need to be further evaluated prior to application in clinical practice, but current data show much promise.

Embryo Cryopreservation

The Human Fertilisation and Embryology Authority (HFEA, 2010) estimated that there were between 15,000 and 20,000 births in the UK from the use of frozen-thawed embryos in 2010. Despite the poor pregnancy rates achieved when transferring frozen embryos (22.8%), which were generally lower than those for fresh embryo transfers (33.4%) (HFEA, 2010), embryo cryopreservation is increasingly being adopted to preserve and protect the fertility of donors who delay childbearing, or who are undergoing aggressive treatments such as chemotherapy, radiotherapy, or surgery (Jain and Paulson, 2006). Additionally, not all embryos created during an IVF cycle are used, and cryopreservation allows patients to choose to save unused embryos for subsequent use (HFEA, 2010).

In stark contrast to its relative effect upon sperm, cryopreservation may increase embryo viability in comparison to embryos obtained from slow cooling (Zhang *et al.*, 2011). In general, embryo cryopreservation is considered beneficial as frozen embryos have been shown to be of better quality (Stern *et al.*, 2012), producing more live births, longer gestational periods and heavier birth weights (Wennerholm *et al.*,2009; Henningsen *et al.*, 2011), all predictive indicators of good health in later life. However, evidence suggests that preserved oocytes are less responsive to activation following sperm fusion/injection (Kim *et al.*, 2011), and have lower fertilisation, implantation and pregnancy potential (Bernard and Fuller., 1996). Cryopreservation also increases the rate of oocyte aneuploidy (Van der Elst *et al.*, 1993; Bernard and Fuller. 1996; Glenister *et al.*, 1987; Kola *et al.*, 1988; Almeida and Bolton 1993;). which could be a dominant factor in poor success rates, and may be linked to the increased risk of Down's Syndrome reported in ART children (Kola *et al.*, 1988).

Nonetheless, research strongly suggests that embryo cryopreservation is not entirely safe (Dulioust *et al.*, 1999; Belva *et al.*, 2008), with some reports suggesting that pre-term births or malformations are more likely in babies born from frozen embryos (Wennerholm, 2000; Alukal and Lipshultz., 2008). This evidence raises concerns regarding the routine use of embryo cryopreservation in ART clinics. Embryo freezing is currently the most commonly used method to preserve patient fertility. However, several alternative options are available to post- and pre-pubertal patients with cancer including oocyte or ovarian tissue cryopreservation for females, and sperm or testicular tissue freezing for males (Jeruss and Woodruff, 2009), all of which merit further investigation and optimisation.

Cryopreservation and Vitrification of Oocytes

To provide more options for pre-pubertal females or single women (with limited waiting-time prior to chemotherapy), a significant body of research has focused upon oocyte freezing (with subsequent *in vitro* maturation of thawed oocytes) and ovarian tissue cryopreservation. The first birth from oocyte freezing was reported in 1986, after which a further 200 offspring have been reported, suggesting that the application of this technique is far from widespread. Fertilisation and cleavage rates following oocyte cryopreservation are satisfactory, yet survival is poor, indicating that much research is required before the technique becomes clinically efficient (Cobo *et al.*, 2011).

In a similar manner to sperm, frozen oocytes are at high risk of cryo-damage and internal organelle deterioration as a result of ice crystal formation, solution effects, and rapid shifts in osmolarity (osmotic shock due to slow-thawing) (Jain and Paulson, 2006). Gualtieri *et al.* (2009) reported that the slow-cooling of human oocytes significantly increased ultrastructural damage involving cortical granule release, mitochondrial injury, and swelling of smooth endoplasmic reticulum vesicles, compared with fresh oocytes. Cryopreservation may also induce disruption of meiotic spindles in oocytes (Gomes *et al.*, 2012). To avoid chromosomal anomalies and aneuploidy, microtubular spindle machinery must function normally during chromosome segregation (into daughter cells) during cellular mitosis and meiosis (Stachecki *et al.*, 2004). Any interruption to the normal function of this apparatus may result in miscarriage or congenital disorders such as ventricular septal defects (Winslow *et al.*, 2001; Gomes *et al.*, 2012).

Reductions of nearly 20% have been observed in cleavage rate and embryo quality of cryopreserved oocytes when compared to fresh oocytes, due to irreversible and permanent damage to meiotic microtubule re-polymerisation (Chamayou *et al.*, 2006). However, more recent studies believe that such disruption is reversible, and that the spindle may be reconstructed naturally following thawing. If this theory is correct, the risk of embryonic aneuploidy in cryopreserved oocytes would be no greater than for fresh oocytes (Gomes *et al.*, 2012). Furthermore, cryopreservation and exposure to certain cryoprotectants such as dimethylsulfoxide (DMSO) and propanediol (PROH), is believed to increase premature cortical granule exocytosis (by 70-80%) in metaphase II (MII) oocytes as a result of transient cryoprotectant-induced and artificial intracellular calcium ion concentration increase (Canovas *et al.*, 2009).

Vitrification is a relatively new cryopreservation technique that facilitates the ultra-rapid freezing of mainly oocytes and blastocysts (Donnez and Dolmans, 2011). There has been a significant increase in live-births, rising from 29.4% before, to 39% after, 2005 as a result of the development of vitrification techniques (Oktay *et al.*, 2006). This has raised hopes in the scientific community that vitrification may replace traditional freezing protocols. Indeed, several studies have reported potential benefits of vitrification in terms of improving oocyte/embryo quality by reducing the potential for cryo-injury (compared with traditional freezing techniques) (Oktay *et al.*, 2006; Wikland *et al.*, 2010; Herrero *et al.*, 2011). However, other reports have identified a much higher risk of spindle defects and chromosome bridging in vitrified blastocysts compared to fresh blastocysts. Consequently, and despite being used more frequently than oocyte slow-freezing, vitrification is still not completely accepted as a cryopreservation technique and further studies are required to determine the potential dangers of vitrification with regard to the more susceptible mitotic phases, and to investigate the potential consequences of abnormal spindles upon chromosome segregation (Chatzimeletiou *et al.*, 2011).

Conclusion and Future Perspectives

Whilst advances in assisted reproductive technology (ART) have revolutionised infertility treatment, success rates vary notably. An increasing body of evidence strongly suggests that routine ART techniques may inadvertently induce detrimental effects upon gametes and embryos, compromising either gamete fertility or embryonic viability. Consequently, it is critical that ART protocols are investigated and refined as necessary to optimise the chance of success.

Iatrogenic damage to gametes and embryos appears to be a relatively common occurrence in ART, and may be reduced considerably by identifying the problems concerned and by modifying or replacing protocols accordingly. Mishaps such as the use of cytotoxic laboratory containers or medium, sub-optimal sperm liquefaction temperature and time, or incubator malfunction, are just some of the basic examples that can lead to compromised success. Investigative research continues to improve success rates and develop novel tests to select the best quality gametes and embryos in terms of implantation success and healthy development. As the number of couples seeking fertility treatment worldwide increases, the efficacy of ART is more important than ever. It is essential that reproductive scientists undertake concerted research efforts to maximise the efficiency of ART protocols, and provide patients with the best chances of success.

References

Aitken, R.J. 1994. A free radical theory of male infertility. *Reprod. Fertil. Dev.* 6, 19-23; discussion 23-4.

Aitken, R.J. 1995. Free radicals, lipid peroxidation and sperm function. *Reprod. Fertil. Dev.* 7, 659-668.

Aitken, R.J., Buckingham, D.W., Brindle, J., Gomez, E., Baker, H.W., Irvine, D.S. 1995. Analysis of sperm movement in relation to the oxidative stress created by leukocytes in washed sperm preparations and seminal plasma. *Hum. Reprod.* 10, 2061-2071.

Aitken, R.J., Gordon, E., Harkiss, D., Twigg, J.P., Milne, P., Jennings, Z., Irvine, D.S. 1998. Relative impact of oxidative stress on the functional competence and genomic integrity of human spermatozoa. *Biol. Reprod.* 59, 1037-1046.

Aitken, R.J., De Iuliis, G.N., McLachlan, R.I. 2009. Biological and clinical significance of DNA damage in the male germ line. *Int. J. Androl.* 32, 46-56.

Allamaneni, S.S., Agarwal, A., Rama, S., Ranganathan, P., Sharma, R.K. 2005. Comparative study on density gradients and swim-up preparation techniques utilizing neat and cryopreserved spermatozoa. *Asian J. Androl.* 7, 86-92.

Almeida, P.A., Bolton, V.N. 1993. Immaturity and chromosomal abnormalities in oocytes that fail to develop pronuclei following insemination in vitro. *Hum. Reprod.* 8, 229-232.

Alikani, M. 2007. The debate surrounding human embryonic stem cell research in the USA. *Reprod. Biomed. Online* 15 (Suppl 2), 7-11.

Alikani, M., Cohen, J., Tomkin, G., Garrisi, G.J., Mack, C., Scott, R.T. 1999. Human embryo fragmentation in vitro and its implications for pregnancy and implantation. *Fertil. Steri.* 71, 836-842.

Alikani, M., Schimmel, T., Willadsen, S.M. 2005. Cytoplasmic fragmentation in activated eggs occurs in the cytokinetic phase of the cell cycle, in lieu of normal cytokinesis, and in response to cytoskeletal disorder. *Mol. Hum. Reprod.* 11, 335-344.

Alukal, J.P., Lipshultz, L.I. 2008. Safety of assisted reproduction, assessed by risk of abnormalities in children born after use of in vitro fertilization techniques. *Nat. Clin. Pract. Urol.* 5, 140-150.

Amor, D.J., Halliday, J. 2008. A review of known imprinting syndromes and their association with assisted reproduction technologies. *Hum. Reprod.* 23, 2826-2834.

Bavister, B.D., 1995. Culture of preimplantation embryos: facts and artifacts. *Hum. Reprod. Update.* 1, 91-148.

Belva, F., Henriet, S., Van Del Abbeel, E., Camus, M., Devroey, P., Van Der Elst, J., Liebaers, I., Haentjens, P., Bonduelle, M. 2008. Neonatal outcome of 937 children born after transfer of cryopreserved embryos obtained by ICSI and IVF and comparison with outcome data of fresh ICSI and IVF cycles. *Hum. Reprod.* 23, 2227-38.

Bernard, A., Fuller, B.J. 1996. Cryopreservation of human oocytes: a review of current problems and perspectives. *Hum. Reprod. Update.* 2, 193-207.

Boomsma, C., Heineman, M., Cohlen, B., Farquhar, C. 2007. Semen preparation techniques for intrauterine insemination. Cochrane Database. *Syst. Rev.* 4.

Borges, E., Rossi, L.M., Locambo de Freitas, C.V., Guilherme, P., Bonetti, T.C.S., Iaconelli, A., Pasqualotto, F.F. 2007. Fertilization and pregnancy outcome after intracytoplasmic injection with fresh or cryopreserved ejaculated spermatozoa. *Fertil. Steril.* 87, 316-320.

Canovas, S., Romar, R., Grullon, L.A., Aviles, M., Coy, P. 2009. Pre-fertilization zona pellucida hardening by different cross-linkers affects IVF in pigs and cattle and improves embryo production in pigs. *Reproduction.* 137, 803.

Cean, A., Bogdan, A.T., Păcală, N., Ivan, A., Ilie, D.E. 2011. Mammalian Oocyte Cryopreservation-Review. *Animal Science and Biotechnologies.* 44, 370-375.

Chamayou, S., Ragolia, C., Alecci, C., Storaci, G., Maglia, E., Russo, E., Guglielmino, A. 2006. Meiotic spindle presence and oocyte morphology do not predict clinical ICSI outcomes: a study of 967 transferred embryos. *Reprod. Biomed. Online.* 13, 661-667.

Chatzimeletiou, K., Morrison, E.E., Panagiotidis, Y., Vanderzwalmen, P., Prapas, N., Prapas, Y., Tarlatzis, B.C., Handyside, A.H. 2011. Cytoskeletal analysis of human blastocysts by confocal laser scanning microscopy following vitrification. *Hum. Reprod.* 27, 106-117.

Cobo, A., Diaz, C. 2011. Clinical application of oocyte vitrification: a systematic review and meta-analysis of randomized controlled trials. *Fertil.Steril.* 96, 277-285.

Collins, J.A., Barnhart, K.T., Schlegel, P.N. 2008. Do sperm DNA integrity tests predict pregnancy with in vitro fertilization? *Fertil. Steril.* 89, 823-831.

Dommering, C.J., van der Hout, A.H., Meijers-Heijboer, H., Marees, T., Moll, A.C., 2012. IVF and retinoblastoma revisited. *Fertil. Steril.* 97, 79-81.

Donnez, J., Dolmans, M.M. 2011. Preservation of fertility in females with haematological malignancy. *Br. J. Haematol.* 154, 175-184.

Drost, J.B., Lee, W.R. 1995. Biological basis of germline mutation: comparisons of spontaneous germline mutation rates among drosophila, mouse, and human. *Environ. Mol. Mutagen.* 25, 48-64.

Dulioust, E., Busnel, M.C., Carlier, M., Roubertoux, P., Aurox, M. 1999. Embryo cryopreservation and development: facts, questions and responsibility. *Hum. Reprod.* 14, 1141-1145.

Edwards, R.G., Fishel, S.B., Cohen, J., Fehilly, C.B., Purdy, J.M., Slater, J.M., Steptoe, P.C., Webster, J.M. 1984. Factors influencing the success of in vitro fertilization for alleviating human infertility. *J. In. Vitro. Fert. Embryo. Transf,* 1, 3-23.

Elder, K., Dale, B. 2011. In-Vitro Fertilization, third ed. Cambridge. UK.

Enciso, M., Sarasa, J., Agarwal, A., Fernández, J.L., Gosálvez, J. 2009. A two-tailed Comet assay for assessing DNA damage in spermatozoa. *Reprod. Biomed. Online.* 18, 609-616.

Enciso, M., Iglesias, M., Galán, I., Sarasa, J., Gosálvez, A., Gosálvez, J. 2011. The ability of sperm selection techniques to remove single-or double-strand DNA damage. *Asian J. Androl.* 13, 764-768.

Farr, S.L., Schieve, L.A., Jamieson, D.J. 2007. Pregnancy loss among pregnancies conceived through assisted reproductive technology, United States, 1999-2002. *Am. J. Epidemiol.* 165, 1380-1388.

Gadea, J., Molla, M., Selles, E., Marco, M.A., Garcia-Vazquez, F.A., Gardon, J.C. 2011. Reduced glutathione content in human sperm is decreased after cryopreservation: Effect of the addition of reduced glutathione to the freezing and thawing extenders. *Cryobiology.* 62, 40-46.

Gardner, D.K., Lane, M., Spitzer, A., Batt, P.A. 1994. Enhanced rates of cleavage and development for sheep zygotes cultured to the blastocyst stage in vitro in the absence of serum and somatic cells: amino acids, vitamins, and culturing embryos in groups stimulate development. *Biol. Reprod.* 50, 390-400.

Glenister, P.H., Wood, M.J., Kirby, C. Whittingham, D.G. 1987. Incidence of chromosome anomalies in first-cleavage mouse embryos obtained from frozen-thawed oocytes fertilized in vitro. *Gamete. Res.* 16, 205-216.

Gomes, C., Merlini, M., Konheim, J., Serafini, P., Motta, E.L.A., Baracat, E.C., Smith, G.D. 2012. Oocyte meiotic-stage-specific differences in spindle depolymerization in response to temperature changes monitored with polarized field microscopy and immunocytochemistry. *Fertil. Steril.* 97, 714-719.

Gosálvez, J., López-Fernández, C., Fernández, J.L., Gouraud, A., Holt, W.V. 2011. Relationships between the dynamics of iatrogenic DNA damage and genomic design in mammalian spermatozoa from eleven species. *Mol. Reprod. Dev.* 78, 951-61.

Gosden, R., Trasler, J., Lucifero, D., Faddy, M. 2003. Rare congenital disorders, imprinted genes, and assisted reproductive technology. *Lancet* 361, 1975-1977.

Grasa, P., Coward, K., Young, C., Parrington, J. 2008. The pattern of localization of the putative oocyte activation factor, phospholipase Czeta, in uncapacitated, capacitated, and ionophore-treated human spermatozoa. *Hum. Reprod.* 23, 2512-2522.

Gualtieri, R., Iaccarino, M., Mollo, V., Prisco, M., Iaccarino, S., Talevi, R. 2009. Slow cooling of human oocytes: ultrastructural injuries and apoptotic status. *Fertil. steril.* 91, 1023-1034.

Guner, J., Jones, C., Kashir, J., Turner, K., Coward, K., 2010. Fertile prospects for human embryology training. *Biologist.* 57, 69-76.

Hammadeh, M.E., Askari, A.S., Georg, T., Rosenbaum, P., Schmidt, W. 1999. Effect of freeze–thawing procedure on chromatin stability, morphological and membrane integrity of human spermatozoa in fertile and subfirtile men. *Int. J. Androl.* 22, 155–162.

Healy, D.L,. Trounson, A.O., Andersen, A.N. 1994. Female infertility: causes and treatment. *Lancet*. 343,1539-1544.

Henningsen, A.K., Pinborg, A., Lidegaard, Ø., Vestergaard, C., Forman, J.L., Andersen, A.N. 2011. Perinatal outcome of singleton siblings born after assisted reproductive technology and spontaneous conception: Danish national sibling-cohort study. *Fertil. Steril.* 95, 959-963.

Herrero, L., Martínez, M., Garcia-Velasco, J.A. 2011. Current status of human oocyte and embryo cryopreservation. *Curr. Opin. Obstet. Gynecol.* 23, 245-250.

HFEA: Latest UK IVF figures – 2009 and 2010 [http://www.hfea.gov.uk/ivf-figures-2006.html] [date accessed: 17th June 2012].

Huang, J.Y.J., Chen, H.Y., Tan, S.L., Chian, R.C. 2006. Effects of osmotic stress and cryoprotectant toxicity on mouse oocyte fertilization and subsequent embryonic development in vitro. *Cell. Preserv. Techn.* 4, 149-160.

Hughes, C.M., Lewis, S., McKelvey-Martin, V.J., Thompson, W. 1998. The effects of antioxidant supplementation during Percoll preparation on human sperm DNA integrity. *Hum. Reprod.* 13, 1240-1247.

Inge, G.B., Brinsden, P.R., Elder, K.T. 2005. Oocyte number per live birth in IVF: were Steptoe and Edwards less wasteful? *Hum. Reprod.* 20, 588-592.

Jackson, R.E., Bormann, C.L., Hassun, P.A., Rocha, A.M., Motta, E.L., Serafini, P.C., Smith, G.D. 2010. *Fertil. Steril.* 94, 2626-2630.

Jain, J.K., Paulson, R.J. 2006. Oocyte cryopreservation. *Fertil. Steril.* 86, 1037-1046.

Jeruss, J.S., Woodruff, T.K. 2009. Preservation of fertility in patients with cancer. *N. Engl. J. Med.* 360, 902-911.

Johnston, S.D., Zee, Y.P., Lopez-Fernandez, C., Gosalvez, J. 2012. The Effect of Chilled Storage and Cryopreservation on the Sperm DNA Fragmentation Dynamics of a Captive Population of Koalas. *J. Androl.* [Epub ahead of print].

Kashir, J., Heindryckx, B., Jones, C., De Sutter, P., Parrington, J., Coward, K. 2010. Oocyte activation phospholipase C zeta and human infertility. *Hum. Reprod. Update* 16, 690-703.

Kashir, J., Heynen, A., Jones, C., Durrans, C., Craig, J., Gadea, J., Turner, K., Parrington, J., Coward, K. 2011. Effects of cryopreservation and density-gradient washing on phospholipase C zeta concentrations in human spermatozoa. *Reprod. Biomed. Online*. 23, 263-267.

Keefe, D.L., Liu, L. 2009. Telomeres and reproductive aging. *Reprod Fertil Dev,* 21, 10-4.

Kim, S.H., Ku, S.Y., Sung, K.C., Kang, M.J., Kim, S.A., Kim, H.S., Oh, S.K., Jee, B.C., Suh, C.S., Choi, Y.M., Kim, J.G., Moon, S.Y. 2006. Simplified EM grid vitrification is a convenient and efficient method for mouse mature oocyte cryopreservation. *Yonsei Med. J.* 47, 399-404.

Kim, B.Y., Yoon, S.Y., Cha, S.K., Kwak, K.H., Fissore, R.A., Parys, J.B., Yoon, T.K., Lee, D.R. 2011. Alterations in calcium oscillatory activity in vitrified mouse eggs impact on egg quality and subsequent embryonic development. *Pflugers. Arch.* 461, 515-526.

Khosla, S., Dean, W., Brown, D., Reik, W., Feil, R. 2001. Culture of preimplantation mouse embryos affects fetal development and the expression of imprinted genes. *Biol. Reprod.* 64, 918-926.

Kobayashi, H., Hiura, H., John, R.M., Sato, A., Otsu, E., Kobayashi, N., Suzuki, R., Suzuki, F., Hayashi, C., Utsunomiya, T., Yaegashi, N., Arima, T. 2009. DNA methylation errors at imprinted loci after assisted conception originate in the parental sperm. *Eur. J. Hum. Genet.* 17, 1582-1591.

Kola, I., Kirby, C., Shaw, J., Davey, A., Trounson, A. 1988. Vitrification of mouse oocytes results in aneuploid zygotes and malformed fetuses. *Teratology.* 38, 467-474.

Kusakabe, H., Szczygiel, M.A., Whittingham, D.G., Yanagimachi, R. 2001. Maintenance of genetic integrity in frozen and freeze-dried mouse spermatozoa. *Proc. Natl. Acad. Sci. U. S. A.* 98, 13501-13506.

Lane, M., Gardner, D.K. 1992. Effect of incubation volume and embryo density on the development and viability of mouse embryos in vitro. *Hum. Reprod.* 7, 558-562.

Lane, M., Gardner, D.K. 2001. Vitrification of mouse oocytes using a nylon loop. *Mol. Reprod. Dev.* 58, 342-347.

Larman, M.G., Katz-Jaffe, M.G., Sheehan, C.B., Gardner, D.K. 2007. 1, 2-Propanediol and the Type of Cryopreservation Procedure Adversely Affect Mouse Oocyte Physiology. *Hum. Reprod.* 22, 250-259.

Ledger, W.L. 2009. Demographics of infertility. *Reprod. Biomed. Online.* 18, Suppl 2, 11-14.

Lee, D.R., Yang, Y.H., Eum, J.H., Seo, J.S., Ko, J.J., Chung, H.M., Yoon, T.K. 2007. Effect of using slush nitrogen (SN2) on development of microsurgically manipulated vitrified/warmed mouse embryos. *Hum. Reprod.* 22, 2509-2514.

Li, L., Le, F., Wang, L.Y., Xu, X.R., Lou, H.Y., Zheng, Y.M., Sheng, J.Z., Huang, H.F., Jin, F. 2011. Normal epigenetic inheritance in mice conceived by in vitro fertilization and embryo transfer. *J. Zhejiang Univ. Sci. B.* 12, 796-804.

Li, Z., Zhou, Y., Liu, R., Lin, H., Liu, W., Xiao, W., Lin, Q. 2011. Effects of semen processing on the generation of reactive oxygen species and mitochondrial membrane potential of human spermatozoa. *Andrologia.* 44, 157-163.

Liu, J.L., Kusakabe, H., Chang, C.C., Suzuki, H., Schmidt, D.W., Julian, M., Pfeffer, R., Bormann, C.L., Tian, X.C., Yanagimachi, R., Yang, X. 2004. Freeze-dried sperm fertilization leads to full-term development in rabbits. *Biol. Reprod.* 70, 1776-1781.

Maher, E.R., Brueton, L.A., Bowdin, S.C., Luharia, A., Cooper, W., Cole. T.R., Macdonald, F., Sampson, J.R., Barratt, C.L., Reik, W., Hawkins, M.M. 2003. Beckwith-Wiedemann syndrome and assisted reproduction technology (ART). *J. Med. Genet.* 40, 62-64.

Maher, E.R. 2005. Imprinting and assisted reproductive technology. *Hum. Mol. Genet.* 14 Spec No 1, R133-8.

Martinez-Soto, J.C., Garcia-Vazquez, F.A., Gumbao, D., Landeras, J., Gadea, J. 2011. Assessment of two thawing processes of cryopreserved human sperm in pellets. *Cryobiology.* 63, 131-136.

Merlob, P., Sapir, O., Sulkes, J., Fisch, B. 2005. The prevalence of major congenital malformations during two periods of time,1986-1994 and 1995-2002 in newborns conceived by assisted reproduction technology. *Eur. J. Med. Genet.* 48, 5-11.

Mitchell, L.A., De Iuliis, G.N., Aitken, R.J. 2011. The TUNEL assay consistently underestimates DNA damage in human spermatozoa and is influenced by DNA compaction and cell vitality: development of an improved methodology. *Int. J. Androl.* 34, 2-13.

Moll, A.C., Imhof, S.M., Schouten-van Meeteren, A.Y., van Leeuwen, F.E. 2003. In-vitro fertilisation and retinoblastoma. *Lancet.* 361, 1392.

Morbeck, D.E., Khan, Z., Barnidge, D.R., Walker, D.L. 2010. Washing mineral oil reduces contaminants and embryotoxicity. *Fertil. Steril.* 94, 2747-2752.

Oktay, K., Cil, A.P., Bang, H., 2006. Efficiency of oocyte cryopreservation: a meta-analysis. *Fertil. Steril.* 86, 70-80.

Olivennes, F., Fanchin, R., Lédée, N., Righini, C., Kadoch, I.J., Frydman, R. 2002. Perinatal outcome and developmental studies on children born after IVF. *Hum. Reprod. Update* 8, 17-128.

Otsuki, J., Nagai, Y., Chiba, K. 2007. Peroxidation of mineral oil used in droplet culture is detrimental to fertilization and embryo development. *Fertil. Steril.* 88, 741-743.

Otsuki, J., Nagai, Y., Chiba, K. 2009. Damage of embryo development caused by peroxidized mineral oil and its association with albumin in culture. *Fertil. Steril.* 91, 1745-1749.

Ozkavukcu, S., Erdemli, E., Isik, A., Oztuna, D., Karahuseyinoglu, S. 2008. Effects of cryopreservation on sperm parameters and ultrastructural morphology of human spermatozoa. *J. Assist. Reprod. Genet.* 25, 403–411.

Pacey, A.A. 2010. Environmental and lifestyle factors associated with sperm DNA damage. *Hum. Fertil. (Camb)* 13, 189-193.

Papi, M., Brunelli, R., Sylla, L., Parasassi, T., Monaci, M., Maulucci, G., Missori, M., Arcovito, G., Ursini, F., De Spirito, M. 2010. Mechanical properties of zona pellucida hardening. *Eur. Biophys. J.* 39, 987-992.

Paria, B.C., Dey, S.K. 1990. Preimplantation embryo development in vitro: cooperative interactions among embryos and role of growth factors. *Proc. Natl. Acad. Sci. U. S. A.* 87, 4756-4760.

Rienzi, L., Vajta, G., Ubaldi, F. 2011. New culture devices in ART. *Placenta.* 32, Suppl 3, S248-51.

Rinaudo, P,. Schultz, R.M. 2004. Effects of embryo culture on global pattern of gene expression in preimplantation mouse embryos. *Reproduction* 128, 301-311.

Robinson , J.J., Wilmut, I., Sinclair, K.D. 2001. Epigenetic change in IGF2R is associated with fetal overgrowth after sheep embryo culture. *Nat. Genet.* 27, 153-154

Schultz, R.M. 2005. From egg to embryo: a peripatetic journey. *Reproduction.* 130, 825-828.

Sharma, R.K., Agarwal, A. 1996. A Sperm quality improvement in cryopreserved human semen. *J. Urol.* 156, 1008-1012.

Shekarriz, M., DeWire, D.M., Thomas, A.J. Jr., Agarwal, A. 1995. A method of human semen centrifugation to minimize the iatrogenic sperm injuries caused by reactive oxygen species. *Eur. Urol.* 28, 31-35.

Silber, S.J., Grudzinskas, G., Gosden, R.G. 2008. Successful pregnancy after microsurgical transplantation of an intact ovary. *N. Engl. J. Med,* 359, 2617-2618.

Smith, G.D., Takayama, S., Swain, J.E. 2012. Rethinking in vitro embryo culture: new developments in culture platforms and potential to improve assisted reproductive technologies. *Biol. Reprod.* 86, 62.

Stachecki, J.J., Munne, S., Cohen, J. 2004. Spindle organization after cryopreservation of mouse, human, and bovine oocytes. *Reprod. Biomed. Online*. 8, 664 –677.

Stern, J.E., Liebermen, E.S., Macaluso, M., Racowsky, C. 2012. Is cryopreservation of embryos a legitimate surrogate marker of embryo quality in studies of assisted reproductive technology conducted using national databases? *Fertil. Steril.* 97, 890-893.

Strömberg , B., Dahlquist, G., Ericson, A., Finnström, O., Köster, M., Stjernqvist, K. 2002. Neurological sequelae in children born after in-vitro fertilisation: a population-based study. *Lancet.* 359, 461-465.

Sutcliffe, A.G., Peters, C.J., Bowdin, S., Temple, K., Reardon, W., Wilson, L., Clayton-Smith, J., Brueton, L.A., Bannister, W., Maher, E.R. 2006. Assisted reproductive therapies and imprinting disorders--a preliminary British survey. *Hum. Reprod.* 21, 1009-1011.

Swann, K., Saunders, C., Rogers, N., Lai, F. 2006. PLC zeta: A sperm protein that triggers Ca2+ oscillations and egg activation in mammals. *Semin. Cell. Dev. Biol.* 17, 264-273.

Tavalaee, M., Deemeh, M.R., Arbabian, M., Nasr-Esfahani, M.H. 2012. Density gradient centrifugation before or after magnetic-activated cell sorting: which technique is more useful for clinical sperm selection? *J. Assisted Reprod. Genet.* 29, 31-38.

Thompson, J.G. 2007. Culture without the petri-dish. *Theriogenology.* 67, 16-20.

Twigg, J., Irvine, D.S., Houston, P., Fulton, N., Michael, L., Aitken, R.J. 1998. Iatrogenic DNA damage induced in human spermatozoa during sperm preparation: protective significance of seminal plasma. *Mol. Hum. Reprod.* 4, 439-445.

Vajta, G., Peura, T.T., Holm. P., Páldi, A., Greve, T., Trounson, A.O., Callesen, H. 2000. New method for culture of zona-included or zona-free embryos: the Well of the Well (WOW) system. *Mol. Reprod. Dev.* 55, 256-264.

Vajta, G., Rienzi, L., Cobo, A., Yovich, J. 2010. Embryo culture: can we perform better than nature? *Reprod. Biomed. Online.* 20, 453-469.

Van der Elst, J., Nerinckx, S., Van Steirteghem, A.C. 1993. Association of ultrarapid freezing of mouse oocytes with increased polyploidy at the pronucleate stage, reduced cell numbers in blastocysts and impaired fetal development. *J. Reprod. Fertil.* 99, 25-32.

Wennerholm, U.B., Söderström-Anttila, V., Bergh, C., Aittomäki, K., Hazekamp, J., Nygren, K.G., Selbing, A., Loft, A. 2009. Children born after cryopreservation of embryos or oocytes: a systematic review of outcome data. *Hum. Reprod.* 24, 2158-2172.

Wennerholm, W.B. 2000. Cryopreservation of embryos and oocytes: obstetric outcome and health in children. *Hum Reprod,* 15 Suppl 5, 18-25.

Wikland, M., Hardarson, T., Hillensjö, T., Westin, C., Westlander, G., Wood, M., Wennerholm, U. 2010. Obstetric outcomes after transfer of vitrified blastocysts. *Hum. Reprod.* 25, 1699-1707.

Winslow, K.L., Yang, D., Blohm, P.L., Brown, S.E., Jossim, P., Nguyen, K. 2001. Oocyte cryopreservation: a three year follow up of sixteen births. *Fertil. Steril.* 76 (Suppl 1), 120 –121.

Younglai, E., Holt, D., Brown, P., Jurisicova, A., Casper, R. 2001. Sperm swim-up techniques and DNA fragmentation. *Hum. Reprod.* 16, 1950-1953.

Zhang, Z., Liu, Y., Xing, Q., Zhou, P. and Cao, Y. 2011. Cryopreservation of human failed-matured oocytes followed by in vitro maturation: vitrification is superior to the slow freezing method. *Reprod. Biol. Endocrinol.* 9, 156.

Zini, A., Mak, V., Phang, D., Jarvi, K. 1999. Potential adverse effect of semen processing on human sperm deoxyribonucleic acid integrity. *Fertil. Steril.* 72, 496-499.

Zini, A., Nam, R.K., Mak, V., Phang, D., Jarvi, K. 2000. Influence of initial semen quality on the integrity of human sperm DNA following semen processing. *Fertil. Steril.* 74, 824-827

Zribi, N., Feki Chakroun, N., El Euch, H., Gargouri, J., Bahloul, A., Ammar Keskes, L. 2010. Effects of cryopreservation on human sperm deoxyribonucleic acid integrity. *Fertil. Steril.* 93, 159-166.

In: Infertility
Editors: R. Nascimento and H. V. Boas
ISBN: 978-1-62257-909-9

Chapter 5

Genetic Factors of Male Infertility

Hideyuki Kobayashi, [1,*] ***Koichi Nagao and Koichi Nakajima***
[1] Department of Urology, Toho University School of Medicine, Tokyo, Japan

Abstract

Our understanding of genomic medicine has increased with developments in molecular biology, stem cell technology, and research on the DNA content of the human genome. Advances in these areas have had considerable impact on the field of genetic male infertility. Many causes of genetic male infertility have been extensively studied, including Klinefelter syndrome (47, XXY), chromosomal aneuploidies, chromosomal translocation, Y-chromosome microdeletions, X-chromosome abnormalities, single-gene defects, and abnormalities in DNA mismatch repair. However, many genetic abnormalities that result in male infertility are still unknown. Indeed, it is likely that most cases of male infertility have a definable underlying genetic cause. A better understanding of the genetic basis of infertility will lead to improvements in its diagnosis and treatment.

Introduction

The field of genomic medicine has grown with advances in molecular medicine, stem cell biology, and the human genome project. The field of genetic male infertility has also benefited from these areas of research. However, most genetic abnormalities do not cause male infertility, which is relatively little studied. It is likely that most currently inexplicable and idiopathic infertility cases are due to genetic causes. Recognized genetic defects are generally divided into five categories. The first category is point mutations in single genes, the second is chromosomal disorders and chromosomal segment abnormalities (deletions, duplications, and aneuploidy), the third is polygenic or multifactorial genetic defects, the

[*] To whom correspondence should be addressed at: Department of Urology, Toho University; School of Medicine, Tokyo, Japan, 6-11-1, Omori-Nishi, Ota-ku, Tokyo 143-8541, Japan; TEL +81-3-3762-4151 FAX +81-3-3768-8817; E-mail: hideyukk@med.toho-u.ac.jp.

fourth is epigenetic modification, and the fifth is mitochondrial disorders. New developments in the genetic causes of male infertility have tremendous implications for the diagnosis and treatment of this condition.

X-Chromosome Abnormalities and Infertility

It has become clear that the X chromosome may be as important as the Y in determining male fertility potential. X-chromosome translocations, partial deletions, and inversions resulting in severe infertility and azoospermia have been reported [1,2,3] [4] [5]. Infertility from structural abnormalities may occur through the direct interruption of a gene at a breakpoint region, or as a consequence of a position effect in which an uninterrupted gene does not function normally because of a change in its chromosomal environment.

A few studies have examined mutations in X-linked genes in male infertility patients [6] [7]. In a study of 56 infertile men with oligozoospermia or azoospermia, mutations in the *SOX3* (sex determining region Y box 3) gene were observed [6]. The mouse homolog of this gene is expressed found in the developing gonad and brain, and when disrupted, causes hypogonadism with a loss of germ cells.

Mutations in the human *FATE* (*Xp28*) gene have also been found in infertile men [7]. This gene encodes a 21-kDa polypeptide that is not related to any known protein. *FATE* is a testis-specific gene expressed in the fetus after sex determination, and co-expressed with SRY in the 7-week-old testis. In a study of the *FATE* gene in 144 randomly chosen infertile men and 100 proven fertile men, 2 *FATE* mutations were found. Each mutation was found only once, and neither was found in the controls. Neither affected patient had a karyotype abnormality or a Y chromosome microdeletion. However, in one affected patient, a maternal uncle also carried the mutation and was fertile. Therefore, *FATE* gene mutations may contribute to male infertility, but their role is still unclear.

The *ZFX* gene, located on the X chromosome, has also been implicated in human infertility [8]. This gene encodes a zinc-finger protein that appears to be a transcriptional activator and may function in spermatogenesis. A mouse study using a reverse genetic strategy and mutation of the mouse homolog, *Zfx,* suggested that the *ZFX* gene has a role in reproduction. Mice carrying a mutated *Zfx* gene showed a decreased primordial germ cell number during the embryonic period. After birth, the mutant mice were smaller, had smaller testes and epididymides, and had half the sperm concentration of wild-type mice [9].

Meiotic Drive and Sexually Antagonistic Genes

It is interesting that a disproportionate number of male-specific genes are found on the X chromosome in mice. Two theories have been offered to explain this phenomenon: meiotic drive and sexually antagonistic genes [10]. Compared with autosomes, sex chromosomes are thought to be more susceptible to meiotic drive, in which there is a preferential transmission of certain alleles to gametes and offspring over their homologs, a phenomenon distinct from the Mendelian pattern. Such a process could skew the transmission of X chromosomes over Y chromosomes, perhaps driven by X-linked genes critical for spermatogenesis.

Alternatively, the theory of sexually antagonistic genes, which is often invoked to explain why the Y chromosome is laden with spermatogenesis genes, may also account for the abundance of male-specific X-chromosome genes. Sexually antagonistic genes may enhance the reproductive strength in one sex and diminish it in the other, and their accumulation on sex chromosomes may occur as follows. If a recessive mutation exists that enhances male reproductive fitness, it would be more likely to have an immediate benefit for males if located on the X chromosome than on an autosome, thus increasing the chance that the allele would permeate the population. Once permeated, female "fitness" might decrease, and adaptive pressures would serve to limit the gene expression to males, thus augmenting the number of critical spermatogenesis genes on the X chromosome [10].

This story becomes even more complicated when we consider that spermatogenesis genes also exist on autosomes. One theory presupposes that autosomal fertility genes arose as "retrogenes" transposed from the X chromosome [11]. The silencing of the X chromosome during male meiosis could create a driving force for the shift of X-linked genes to autosomes to preserve the expression of critical genes required for germ-cell development. It appears that many such retrogenes, i.e., genes that lack introns that are present in their progenitors, originated from X-linked progenitor genes and are specifically expressed in the testis [11]. Thus, the X chromosome is likely to be important for understanding human male infertility.

Chromosomal Aneuploidies

Klinefelter Syndrome

A genetic anomaly is thought to be responsible for 10% of non-obstructive azoospermia (NOA) cases, and Klinefelter syndrome (KS; 47, XXY), which occurs in 1/500 to 1/1000 live births, is the most common known genetic cause of nonobstructive azoospermia. This syndrome is described by a triad of findings: small and firm testes, azoospermia, and gynecomastia. Other features include increased height, decreased intelligence, varicosities, obesity, diabetes, and an increased likelihood of extragonadal germ cell tumors, leukemia, and breast cancer. Most affected individuals, however, do not exhibit the classic clinical phenotype.

Most KS cases are nonmosaic, with all the cells demonstrating a 47, XXY genotype. When mosaicism does occur, a variable percentage of 46, XY cells is mixed with the 47, XXY cells. The additional X, through an unknown mechanism, sets events in motion that lead to many disparate features of KS, from androgenic and spermatogenic failure to difficulties in expressive language learning [12]. In addition, follicle stimulating hormone (FSH) and luteinizing hormone (LH) are elevated, demonstrating a compensatory output in response to the damaged spermatogenic and androgenic cells and functions of the testes [13] [14]. As a result, patients with KS exhibit severe oligozoospermia or azoospermia, and low testosterone.

Even though a patient may show no sperm in the ejaculate, testicular sperm extraction (TESE) successfully finds spermatozoa in up to 69% of KS men, and this sperm can be used in conjunction with intracytoplasmic sperm injection (ICSI) to effect fertilization, embryo development, and term pregnancy [15] [16,17]. Many live births of 46, XY or 46, XX children following this procedure have been reported [18] [19] [20].

Y-Chromosome Microdeletions

The detailed molecular geography of the Y chromosome is important for understanding the clinical consequences of Y-chromosomal microdeletions that eliminate genes that may be necessary or helpful for optimal spermatogenesis. The human Y chromosome has a long arm (Yq) and a short arm (Yp). The euchromatic portion of Yq includes eight palindromic sequences, with P8 closest to the centromere and P1 the most distal. The ends of these arms are known as pseudoautosomal regions, and the long segment between them is called the male-specific Y (MSY) region. The MSY region contains many of the genes necessary for spermatogenesis, and is unique in the human genome [22]. For example, *SRY*, located on Yp, is an essential member of the cascade of genes that ultimately determines the fate of the bipotential gonad [21]. In individuals with Y-chromosome microdeletions, nearly the entire MSY region is absent from the genome; consequently, there is no spermatogenesis. Karyotype analysis is prognostic and definitive in these cases, eliminating the need for testis biopsy or TESE. Thus, karyotype analysis should be performed in all NOA patients before any surgical intervention.

In the 1970s, Tiepolo and Zuffardi reported that a grossly intact Y chromosome is important for spermatogenesis to occur, and proposed the existence of regions of necessity, termed azoospermia factors (AZF) [23]. As the molecular structure of the Y chromosome was being elucidated in the mid-1990s, three specific microdeletions of significant clinical frequency were detected and described in men with sperm-production deficiency. The original acronyms for these three microdeleted regions was derived from that suggested by Tiepolo and Zuffardi, when it was thought that each was spatially and topographically distinct [23]. It is now known that the AZFa region stands on its own, while the original AZFb and AZFc microdeletions represent just two possible microdeletions of the many that can occur within one stretch of the MSY, with a proximal endpoint located in P5 and distal endpoint in P1; AZFb and AZFc overlap. In men with NOA or severe oligozoospermia, a Y-chromosome microdeletion assay should be performed prior to tissue extraction to search for sperm or using ejaculated sperm to attempt fertilization.

Microdeletion of the AZFa region occurs in approximately 1% of NOA men, and although the molecular anatomy of this region does not involve any of the eight palindromes, if the AZFa region is deleted, spermatozoa will not be found upon TESE [24] [25]. The AZFb or AZFb/c microdeletion is found in 1-3% of NOA men. In these cases, there is little chance that sperm will be retrievable from the testis tissue [25]. The AZFc microdeletion is the most common, present in 1 in 4000 men overall, 13% of NOA males, and 6% of severely oligospermic men [26] [27]. Most men with AZFc microdeletion present with NOA or severe oligozoospermia and consequent sterility or infertility [28]. The spectrum of spermatogenic deficiency is a tight one, ranging from no spermatozoa found on TESE to markedly reduced numbers of sperm in the ejaculate. In the 42 men with AZFc microdeletion reported, 62% were azoospermic (although sperm was obtained from two-thirds of these subjects upon subsequent TESE), and 38% were severely oligospermic. Therefore, 81% had spermatozoa that could be used in conjunction with ICSI to try to achieve fertility, and 19% of the subjects had no sperm available from either the ejaculate or testis tissue.

These findings highlight the need for a karyotype and Y-chromosomal microdeletion assay as complementary tests in all NOA and severely oligozoospermic men, prior to obtaining ejaculated or testicular sperm and performing ICSI. The results of these tests are informative to optimize the prognosis and family planning for these patients.

Other Structural Anomalies

Many other important structural anomalies involving the Y chromosome may be found in the karyotypic analysis of infertile males [29]. The ring Y (r(Y)), results from the circularization of a Y chromosome in which the terminal ends of the chromosome have been lost, and the arms of the chromosomes have fused [30]. Most such cases present as mosaics (46, X, r(Y)/45, X), and the phenotype is variable, ranging from Turner syndrome to normal male external genitalia with azoospermia. The phenotype depends not only on the percentage of cells that contain r(Y) but also on the amount of chromosomal material lost [31]. Other Y-chromosome abnormalities include isodicentric Y (two short arms, two centromeres, and a fused, truncated long arm), truncated Y, and various mosaic states with 45, X cells [32].

Structural chromosomal aberrations of autosomes include Robertsonian and reciprocal (non-Robertsonian) translocations [33]. Reciprocal and Robertsonian translocations (in which material from chromosomes 13, 14, 15, 21, and 22 are involved in as many as 15 different translocations) are at least eight times more common in infertile men than in unselected newborn males. Carriers of Robertsonian translocations are at particular risk for pregnancies that miscarry and for offspring with mental retardation and birth defects. In addition, autosomal inversions, particularly those involving chromosome 9, are eight times more likely to occur in infertile than in fertile men, although no phenotype is associated with these inversions [32].

Other Sex Chromosome Aneuploidies

XYY syndrome can also result in infertility. Men with 47, XYY may be taller than average, have decreased intelligence, a higher risk for leukemia, and may exhibit aggressive or antisocial behavior [34] [35]. Semen analysis can show severe oligozoospermia or azoospermia. In addition, elevated FSH, with normal testosterone and LH, is seen in these men. In azoospermic XYY men, testis biopsies demonstrate maturation arrest or Sertoli cells-only.

XX male syndrome generally presents with gynecomastia at puberty or with azoospermia [36]. Affected men have normal external and internal genitalia, but hormone evaluation reveals elevated FSH and LH and low to normal testosterone levels. Testicular pathology reveals absent spermatogenesis with hyalinization of seminiferous tubules, fibrosis, and Leydig cell clumping.

Kallmann Syndrome

Kallmann syndrome is a type of hypogonadotropic hypogonadism (HH) that results from a failure of GnRH-releasing neurons to migrate to the olfactory lobe during development. There are X-linked, autosomal-dominant, and autosomal-recessive forms of HH [37], and Kallmann syndrome represents the most common X-linked HH disorder in male infertility. A mutation in the X-linked *KAL1* gene, which encodes anosmin 1, a neural cell adhesion glycoprotein found in some embryonic extracellular matrices, is the basis for the sex-linked form of the disease. Less commonly, structural chromosomal defects resulting in the loss of regions of the X chromosome may encompass the *KAL1* gene, resulting in a genomic form of familial X-linked Kallmann syndrome [38]. In addition, autosomal dominant (KAL2) and recessive (KAL3) transmission of Kallmann syndrome have been reported [39] [40].

Because of the lack of GnRH, patients with Kallmann syndrome present with no serum gonadotropins, small, nonfunctioning testes, and a short penis. The puberty of these patients is delayed. Although infertility may represent the only phenotypic abnormality, anosmia may be present due to developmental failure of the olfactory bulb. In some cases, congenital deafness, asymmetry of the cranium and face, cleft palate, cerebellar dysfunction, cryptorchidism, or renal abnormalities are present. Hormone replacement is necessary, and spermatogenesis and subsequent fertility occur with coordinated gonadotropin stimulation [41]. The infertility is treatable with gonadotropin replacement for 12 to 18 months [42,43].

Congenital Bilateral Absence of the Vas Deferens (CBAVD)

CBAVD is found in 1% of infertile males and in up to 6% of those with obstructive azoospermia [44] [45]. Patients with CBAVD have normal testes and consistency, as spermatogenesis is unaffected. However, the vasa are absent bilaterally, which can be assessed by palpation. CBAVD has two genetic etiologies: one involves mutations in the same genes that underlie cystic fibrosis, and the other involves unknown genetic mechanisms controlling mesonephric duct differentiation [46,47].

Most cases of CBAVD result from mutations in the maternal and paternal copies of the *CFTR* gene, which encodes the cystic fibrosis transmembrane conductance regulator (CFTR) protein. Mutations in the *CFTR* gene represent the most common autosomal recessive disease. CFTR is crucial for maintaining the viscosity and fluidity of epithelial secretions by regulating the sodium/chloride balance. Clinical disease is determined by the combination of mutations of *CFTR* alleles. Two mild mutations may result in only CBAVD if the individual is male, while two severe mutations, each dramatically altering the function or quantity of CFTR, will lead to clinical cystic fibrosis (CF). CF patients have chronic pulmonary obstruction and infection, pancreatic insufficiency, neonatal meconium ileus, and infertility.

Androgen Insensitivity Syndromes

Androgen insensitivity syndromes are defined as complete, partial, and minimal.

Complete Androgen Insensitivity

Genotypic 46, XY individuals who lack a functional androgen receptor (AR) display complete androgen insensitivity syndrome. This syndrome can be due to AR gene deletion, but more commonly results from point mutations in the gene that cause a loss of function of the protein. Individuals with this syndrome are pseudohermaphrodites who display an unambiguously female appearance. Female external genitalia develop because, despite high circulating testosterone levels, the tissues are resistant to androgen action. Thus, DHT-dependent masculinization of the external genital primordia is absent. The uterus, ovaries and fallopian tubes are absent in these individuals.

Partial Androgen Insensitivity

The androgen receptor mutation in these patients impairs or changes the receptor function to varying degrees. These patients exhibit a range of congenital genitourinary defects of varying severity, including hypospadias, microphallus, cryptorchidism, gynecomastia, and infertility. At one extreme, the external genitalia resemble those of a nearly normal female phenotype, except for clitoromegaly and/or posterior labial fusion. At the other extreme, the genitalia may resemble those of a morphologically normal male, but the scrotum or phallus may be small, or there may be simple coronal hypospadias or a prominent midline raphe of the scrotum. Reifenstein first reported this syndrome in the 1940s [48].

Minimal Androgen Insensitivity

Individuals with minimal androgen insensitivity exhibit infertility, azoospermia, micropenis, or gynecomastia [49] [50]. Simply put, some mutations vary the AR function in a manner analogous to a rheostat, causing mild functional deficiencies that in some cases can be overcome with increased levels of androgen [51].

Defects in the Gonadotropins and their Receptors

FSH and LH are two key hormones produced by the testis that are necessary for male reproductive function. These gonadotropins are dimeric molecules composed of an α subunit common also to human chorionic gonadotropin (hCG) and thyroid-stimulating hormone (TSH). The β subunits differ and provide the specificity of action.

Mutations in FSH and LH Subunits

Mutations in the FSH and LH subunits can underlie male infertility. The phenotypes vary from complete virilization failure to less severe forms of hypogonadism. Because LH acts on the Leydig cells to stimulate androgen production, LH defects cause androgen deficiency, with its associated developmental and functional features [52]. Deficiencies in FSH occur in subfertile males. Although FSH β-subunit mutations have been suggested, they are rarely found in infertile men [53].

LH and FSH Receptors

The LH and FSH receptors mediate the actions of these gonadotropins in the Leydig and Sertoli cells. Gene mutations causing LH receptor deficiency are rare in humans, but targeted deletion of the LH receptor in the mouse results in male infertility, and the mice display the anatomical features of hypogonadism [54]. In contrast, constitutive activation of the LH receptor leads to precocious male pseudopuberty (but not infertility later in life), whereas pseudohermaphroditism and Leydig cell agenesis are the clinical phenotypes of LH resistance [55] [56]. On the other hand, less is known about the FSH receptors; a mutation has been reported in a hypophysectomized man who is fertile, but the incidence in men is rare [57] [58].

Conclusion

Developments in genomic medicine are expected to elucidate much of the currently unexplained male infertility. With rapid advances in our understanding of male genetic infertility, genetic counseling and testing will likewise improve and have more value than ever before for patients considering assisted reproduction.

Acknowledgments

This study was supported in part by a Grant-in-Aid for Young Scientists (B) of the Japan Society for the Promotion of Science (JSPS) and Grant of Strategic Research Foundation Grant-aided Project for Private schools at Heisei 23th from Ministry of Education, Culture, Sports, Science and Technology of Japan, 2011-2015.

References

[1] Mattei MG, Mattei JF, Ayme S, Giraud F. X-autosome translocations: cytogenetic characteristics and their consequences. *Hum Genet,* 1982 61, 295-309.

[2] Madan K (1983) Balanced structural changes involving the human X: effect on sexual phenotype. *Hum Genet* 63: 216-221.

[3] Cantu JM, Diaz M, Moller M, Jimenez-Sainz M, Sandoval L, et al. (1985) Azoospermia and duplication 3qter as distinct consequences of a familial t(X;3) (q26;q13.2). *Am J Med Genet* 20: 677-684.

[4] Nemeth AH, Gallen IW, Crocker M, Levy E, Maher E (2002) Klinefelter-like phenotype and primary infertility in a male with a paracentric Xq inversion. *J Med Genet* 39: E28.

[5] Lee S, Lee SH, Chung TG, Kim HJ, Yoon TK, et al. (2003) Molecular and cytogenetic characterization of two azoospermic patients with X-autosome translocation. *J Assist Reprod Genet* 20: 385-389.

[6] Raverot G, Lejeune H, Kotlar T, Pugeat M, Jameson JL (2004) X-linked sex-determining region Y box 3 (SOX3) gene mutations are uncommon in men with idiopathic oligoazoospermic infertility. *J Clin Endocrinol* Metab 89: 4146-4148.

[7] Olesen C, Silber J, Eiberg H, Ernst E, Petersen K, et al. (2003) Mutational analysis of the human FATE gene in 144 infertile men. *Hum Genet* 113: 195-201.

[8] Schneider-Gadicke A, Beer-Romero P, Brown LG, Mardon G, Luoh SW, et al. (1989) Putative transcription activator with alternative isoforms encoded by human ZFX gene. *Nature* 342: 708-711.

[9] Luoh SW, Bain PA, Polakiewicz RD, Goodheart ML, Gardner H, et al. (1997) Zfx mutation results in small animal size and reduced germ cell number in male and female mice. *Development* 124: 2275-2284.

[10] Wang PJ, McCarrey JR, Yang F, Page DC (2001) An abundance of X-linked genes expressed in spermatogonia. *Nat Genet* 27: 422-426.

[11] Wang PJ (2004) X chromosomes, retrogenes and their role in male reproduction. *Trends Endocrinol Metab* 15: 79-83.

[12] Visootsak J, Graham JM, Jr. (2006) Klinefelter syndrome and other sex chromosomal aneuploidies. *Orphanet J Rare Dis* 1: 42.

[13] Tomasi PA, Oates R, Brown L, Delitala G, Page DC (2003) The pituitary-testicular axis in Klinefelter's syndrome and in oligo-azoospermic patients with and without deletions of the Y chromosome long arm. *Clin Endocrinol* (Oxf) 59: 214-222.

[14] Aksglaede L, Andersson AM, Jorgensen N, Jensen TK, Carlsen E, et al. (2007) Primary testicular failure in Klinefelter's syndrome: the use of bivariate luteinizing hormone-testosterone reference charts. *Clin Endocrinol* (Oxf) 66: 276-281.

[15] Denschlag D, Tempfer C, Kunze M, Wolff G, Keck C (2004) Assisted reproductive techniques in patients with Klinefelter syndrome: a critical review. *Fertil Steril* 82: 775-779.

[16] Gonsalves J, Turek PJ, Schlegel PN, Hopps CV, Weier JF, et al. (2005) Recombination in men with Klinefelter syndrome. *Reproduction* 130: 223-229.

[17] Schiff JD, Palermo GD, Veeck LL, Goldstein M, Rosenwaks Z, et al. (2005) Success of testicular sperm extraction [corrected] and intracytoplasmic sperm injection in men with Klinefelter syndrome. *J Clin Endocrinol* Metab 90: 6263-6267.

[18] Bourne H, Stern K, Clarke G, Pertile M, Speirs A, et al. (1997) Delivery of normal twins following the intracytoplasmic injection of spermatozoa from a patient with 47,XXY Klinefelter's syndrome. *Hum Reprod* 12: 2447-2450.

[19] Hinney B, Guttenbach M, Schmid M, Engel W, Michelmann HW (1997) Pregnancy after intracytoplasmic sperm injection with sperm from a man with a 47,XXY Klinefelter's karyotype. *Fertil Steril* 68: 718-720.

[20] Komori S, Horiuchi I, Hamada Y, Hasegawa A, Kasumi H, et al. (2004) Birth of healthy neonates after intracytoplasmic injection of ejaculated or testicular spermatozoa from men with nonmosaic Klinefelter's syndrome: a report of 2 cases. *J Reprod Med* 49: 126-130.

[21] Wilhelm D, Palmer S, Koopman P (2007) Sex determination and gonadal development in mammals. *Physiol Rev* 87: 1-28.

[22. Skaletsky H, Kuroda-Kawaguchi T, Minx PJ, Cordum HS, Hillier L, et al. (2003) The male-specific region of the human Y chromosome is a mosaic of discrete sequence classes. *Nature* 423: 825-837.

[23] Tiepolo L, Zuffardi O (1976) Localization of factors controlling spermatogenesis in the nonfluorescent portion of the human Y chromosome long arm. *Hum Genet* 34: 119-124.

[24] Blagosklonova O, Fellmann F, Clavequin MC, Roux C, Bresson JL (2000) AZFa deletions in Sertoli cell-only syndrome: a retrospective study. *Mol Hum Reprod* 6: 795-799.

[25] Hopps CV, Mielnik A, Goldstein M, Palermo GD, Rosenwaks Z, et al. (2003) Detection of sperm in men with Y chromosome microdeletions of the AZFa, AZFb and AZFc regions. *Hum Reprod* 18: 1660-1665.

[26] Reijo R, Lee TY, Salo P, Alagappan R, Brown LG, et al. (1995) Diverse spermatogenic defects in humans caused by Y chromosome deletions encompassing a novel RNA-binding protein gene. *Nat Genet* 10: 383-393.

[27] Reijo R, Alagappan RK, Patrizio P, Page DC (1996) Severe oligozoospermia resulting from deletions of azoospermia factor gene on Y chromosome. *Lancet* 347: 1290-1293.

[28] Kuhnert B, Gromoll J, Kostova E, Tschanter P, Luetjens CM, et al. (2004) Case report: natural transmission of an AZFc Y-chromosomal microdeletion from father to his sons. *Hum Reprod* 19: 886-888.

[29] Faure AK, Aknin-Seifer I, Satre V, Amblard F, Devillard F, et al. (2007) Fine mapping of re-arranged Y chromosome in three infertile patients with non-obstructive azoospermia/cryptozoospermia. *Hum Reprod* 22: 1854-1860.

[30] Arnedo N, Nogues C, Bosch M, Templado C (2005) Mitotic and meiotic behaviour of a naturally transmitted ring Y chromosome: reproductive risk evaluation. *Hum Reprod* 20: 462-468.

[31] Hsu LY (1994) Phenotype/karyotype correlations of Y chromosome aneuploidy with emphasis on structural aberrations in postnatally diagnosed cases. *Am J Med Genet* 53: 108-140.

[32] Van Assche E, Bonduelle M, Tournaye H, Joris H, Verheyen G, et al. (1996) Cytogenetics of infertile men. *Hum Reprod* 11 Suppl 4: 1-24; discussion 25-26.

[33] Yoshida A, Miura K, Shirai M (1997) Cytogenetic survey of 1,007 infertile males. *Urol Int* 58: 166-176.

[34] Walzer S, Gerald PS (1975) Social class and frequency of XYY and XXY. *Science* 190: 1228-1229.

[35] Palanduz S, Aktan M, Ozturk S, Tutkan G, Cefle K, et al. (1998) 47,XYY karyotype in acute myeloid leukemia. *Cancer Genet Cytogenet* 106: 76-77.

[36] Schweikert HU, Weissbach L, Leyendecker G, Schwinger E, Wartenberg H, et al. (1982) Clinical, endocrinological, and cytological characterization of two 46, XX males. *J Clin Endocrinol Metab* 54: 745-752.

[37] Tsai PS, Gill JC (2006) Mechanisms of disease: Insights into X-linked and autosomal-dominant Kallmann syndrome. *Nat Clin Pract Endocrinol Metab* 2: 160-171.

[38] Hershkovitz E, Loewenthal N, Peretz A, Parvari R (2008) Testicular expressed genes are missing in familial X-Linked Kallmann syndrome due to two large different deletions in daughter's X chromosomes. *Horm Res* 69: 276-283.

[39] Dode C, Levilliers J, Dupont JM, De Paepe A, Le Du N, et al. (2003) Loss-of-function mutations in FGFR1 cause autosomal dominant Kallmann syndrome. *Nat Genet* 33: 463-465.

[40] Oliveira LM, Seminara SB, Beranova M, Hayes FJ, Valkenburgh SB, et al. (2001) The importance of autosomal genes in Kallmann syndrome: genotype-phenotype correlations and neuroendocrine characteristics. *J Clin Endocrinol Metab* 86: 1532-1538.

[41] Sigman M (1991) Assisted reproductive technics for the treatment of male factor infertility. *R I Med J* 74: 591-596.

[42] Bhasin S, Ma K, Sinha I, Limbo M, Taylor WE, et al. (1998) The genetic basis of male infertility. *Endocrinol Metab Clin North Am* 27: 783-805, viii.

[43] Layman LC, Cohen DP, Jin M, Xie J, Li Z, et al. (1998) Mutations in gonadotropin-releasing hormone receptor gene cause hypogonadotropic hypogonadism. Nat Genet 18: 14-15.

[44] Ferlin A, Raicu F, Gatta V, Zuccarello D, Palka G, et al. (2007) Male infertility: role of genetic background. *Reprod Biomed Online* 14: 734-745.

[45] Grangeia A, Niel F, Carvalho F, Fernandes S, Ardalan A, et al. (2004) Characterization of cystic fibrosis conductance transmembrane regulator gene mutations and IVS8 poly(T) variants in Portuguese patients with congenital absence of the vas deferens. *Hum Reprod* 19: 2502-2508.

[46] McCallum T, Milunsky J, Munarriz R, Carson R, Sadeghi-Nejad H, et al. (2001) Unilateral renal agenesis associated with congenital bilateral absence of the vas deferens: phenotypic findings and genetic considerations. *Hum Reprod* 16: 282-288.

[47] Southern KW (2007) Cystic fibrosis and formes frustes of CFTR-related disease. *Respiration* 74: 241-251.

[48] Reifenstein EC, Jr. (1947) Hereditary familial hypogonadism. *Proc Am Fed Clin Res* 3: 86.

[49] Aiman J, Griffin JE, Gazak JM, Wilson JD, MacDonald PC (1979) Androgen insensitivity as a cause of infertility in otherwise normal men. *N Engl J Med* 300: 223-227.

[50] Larrea F, Benavides G, Scaglia H, Kofman-Alfaro S, Ferrusca E, et al. (1978) Gynecomastia as a familial incomplete male pseudohermaphroditism type 1: a limited androgen resistance syndrome. *J Clin Endocrinol* Metab 46: 961-970.

[51] McPhaul MJ, Marcelli M, Tilley WD, Griffin JE, Isidro-Gutierrez RF, et al. (1991) Molecular basis of androgen resistance in a family with a qualitative abnormality of the androgen receptor and responsive to high-dose androgen therapy. *J Clin Invest* 87: 1413-1421.

[52] Huhtaniemi I (2000) The Parkes lecture. Mutations of gonadotrophin and gonadotrophin receptor genes: what do they teach us about reproductive physiology? *J Reprod Fertil* 119: 173-186.

[53] Layman LC, Porto AL, Xie J, da Motta LA, da Motta LD, et al. (2002) FSH beta gene mutations in a female with partial breast development and a male sibling with normal puberty and azoospermia. *J Clin Endocrinol* Metab 87: 3702-3707.

[54] Lei ZM, Mishra S, Zou W, Xu B, Foltz M, et al. (2001) Targeted disruption of luteinizing hormone/human chorionic gonadotropin receptor gene. *Mol Endocrinol* 15: 184-200.

[55] Wu SM, Hallermeier KM, Laue L, Brain C, Berry AC, et al. (1998) Inactivation of the luteinizing hormone/chorionic gonadotropin receptor by an insertional mutation in Leydig cell hypoplasia. *Mol Endocrinol* 12: 1651-1660.

[56] Wu RH, Rosenfeld R, Fukushima D (1984) Hypogonadism and Leydig cell hypoplasia unresponsive to human luteinizing hormone (hLH). *Am J Med Sci* 287: 23-25.

[57] Gromoll J, Simoni M, Nordhoff V, Behre HM, De Geyter C, et al. (1996) Functional and clinical consequences of mutations in the FSH receptor. *Mol Cell Endocrinol* 125: 177-182.

[58] Song GJ, Park YS, Lee HS, Kang IS, Lee HK, et al. (2001) Mutation screening of the FSH receptor gene in infertile men. *Mol Cells* 12: 292-297.

In: Infertility
Editors: R. Nascimento and H. V. Boas
ISBN: 978-1-62257-909-9

Chapter 6

Animal Models for Studying Female Infertility

Paloma Sánchez-Aparicio*
Clínica de Medicina de la Reproducción y Ginecología, FivMadrid, Madrid, Spain

Abstract

Female reproductive dysfunction accounts for about 40% of all human infertility cases. Although the molecular aspects of these disorders are still to be determined, the use of animal models over the last decade has shown itself to be a powerful tool in the understanding of female infertility. The development of knock-out and transgenic technology in the last few years has generated more than 300 different mice models that display reproductive defects. In the context of the study of female reproductive biology, the analysis of knock-out and transgenic mice has strongly contributed to clarify the underlying processes leading to follicular development, oocyte maturation, fertilization events or embryo implantation. This chapter provides a comprehensive compilation of the most relevant studies published in this area, from the early pioneering studies to the most recent developments, highlighting how the use of animal models can help us to understand the female reproductive system and the etiology of some female infertile disorders.

Introduction

The standard definition of human infertility is the failure to conceive a pregnancy after a year of unprotected intercourse. According to recent epidemiological studies, one out of every ten couples experiences this problem (Boivin et al. 2007) although the cause of infertility remains unknown in 25% of these cases.

From the analysis of the origin of the problem when this can be determined, we know that around 40% of all human infertility cases correspond to female reproductive dysfunction. Many factors may account for female infertility such as uterine abnormalities, ovarian

* E-mail: aparicio.fiv@gmail.com.

dysfunction, hormonal imbalances, bilateral tubal oclusion, endometriosis, or infections, although infertility is in many cases of unknown etiology.

Commonly, female reproductive success depends on the growth of the ovarian functional units named follicles. Ovaries contain numerous of these units, each one formed by an oocyte, arrested in meiotic prophase I, surrounded by a single layer of granulosa cells. From birth to puberty, follicles remain in a resting state after which a cohort of them receives the adequate signalling for activation, leading to the follicular development first and then to the ovulation event.

This process depends on complex interactions between the ovary and the extra-ovarian environment together with intra-ovarian control. All of them, endocrine, paracrine and autocrine regulatory mechanisms, are mediated by soluble factors belonging to several families of hormones, cytokines or growth factors. In addition, the folliculogenesis is also controlled by mechanisms of cell adhesion, including cell to cell and cell to extracellular matrix interactions; and cellular communication via gap junctions-specialized intercellular channels allowing the free passage of ions and small molecules between adjacent cells-.

All together, these mechanisms of regulation ensure follicle activation, follicle dominance and survival, oocyte resumption of meiosis and growth/differentiation of the companion granulosa cells. Ovulation necessarily requires that the mature follicle rises to the surface of the ovary and that the granulosa cells express the receptors for the luteinizing hormone (LH). Upon ovulation, the empty follicle becomes the corpus luteum and the mature oocyte is transported from the ovary to the uterus through the fallopian tube. Normal ovarian function requires complex interactions between endocrine and paracrine factors. It must be noticed that the follicle is the major functional unit in the ovary and that folliculogenesis allows oocyte growth and maturation coordinated with the somatic cells around, not only the granulosa cells but also theca cells.

Additionally, for pregnancy to occur, successful oocyte fertilization and embryo implantation processes are mandatory. The capacity of a mature oocyte to support fertilization, as well as the subsequent embryo preimplantation and implantation process depends on intrinsic oocyte quality. Indeed, oocytes have already acquired developmental competence along folliculogenesis, and bi-directional communication between the oocyte and its surrounding cells is now widely accepted to be essential for oocyte quality. Following fertilization, the zygote undergoes several divisions and the implantation process allows the resulting embryo to intimately interact with the maternal tissue. At the time of implantation, the uterus must develop into a state that permits embryo attachment in a coordinated way involving hormones produced by the corpus luteum. Unfortunately, a failure of the embryo to implant in a proper way results in growth defects and death of the embryo.

As a result of the extreme complexity of the mechanisms leading to the achievement of pregnancy, several failures, as an inadequate follicular development, ovulation defects, damage at fallopian tube level, poor quality of oocytes or an aberrant implantation process can disturb or block the subsequent reproductive process. Despite the still high incidence of infertility, in the last decade the diagnosis and treatment of female infertility has made enormous progress. The scientific and technological development has made Assisted Reproduction Techniques (ART) possible, and therefore, the management of infertile disorders. This kind of technology combines the use of hormonal therapy with several procedures and techniques such as intrauterine insemination (IUI), in vitro fertilization (FIV/ICSI), embryo transfer or even oocyte donation to ensure reproductive success.

Knockout and Transgenic Mice as Animal Models

For decades researchers have been using animal models like sheep, cows, rats and in particular mice, as a tool to study several human pathologies. This is not strange since despite the fact that there is still a long way from mice to humans both share many genes.

In the 80's, the generation of transgenic mice appeared as a new technology to study the function of specific genes. Upon the injection of genetic material into the pronucleus of fertilized mice oocytes, these oocytes are transferred to the oviduct of pseudopregnant females which are allowed to come to term. Transgenic mice are then born carrying this genetic material incorporated into a non-specific location of their genome. This is the reason why mouse lines carrying the same so-called *transgene* may still display a variety of phenotypes.

In contrast, knockout mice carry the inserted gene at a precise location in the mouse genome. Therefore, it is possible to replace, or *knock out*, a gene with an inactive allele. This technique has become a very powerful tool to determine gene roles and their involvement in diseases. Gene targeting requires a vector and embryonic stem cells as target cells for the vector insertion. In order to determine the function of a specific gene, this must be removed or knocked out in an embryonic stem cell which is then transferred into a recently fertilized embryo. The manipulated cell develops later into different tissues. Finally, the result is a mouse with some cells developed from the knocked out embryonic stem cells.

Mouse models knocking out the activity of a gene provide valuable information about its function, and therefore, contribute to understand how an identical or similar gene may be related to a specific human disease. However, knock out mice technology have some limitations because around 15 % of gene knockouts are developmentally lethal. In addition, the genetically altered mice may fail to produce an observable change. In some cases, and despite these limitations, scientists have succeeded in the identification of specific DNA mutations in humans with particular disorders, and further modelling of the same genetic alteration in mice showing the essential role of a particular gene in a certain process.

Knockout mice compatible with viability and primarily affected on their female reproductive system are described in a number of pioneering studies. Stewart *et al.* in 1992 reported that embryo implantation failed in female mice lacking a functional leukaemia inhibitory factor gene (LIF) indicating that for successful implantation the transient expression of LIF is essential. One year later, Lubahn *et al.* (1993) generated mutant mice by disrupting the estrogen receptor. Female mice resulted unable to respond to estradiol (E_2) although they displayed a normal gross external phenotype, hypoplastic uteri and hyperaemic ovaries. In 1994, Colledge *et al.* published that the oocytes of mutant females for c-mos, a proto-oncogen coding for a kinase implicated in meiotic process, failed to arrest meiosis displaying a reduced fertility; while in 1995, Leonardsson *et al.* reported a significant reduction of ovulation efficiency in mice lacking both tissue-type and urokinase-type Plasminogen Activator (tPA and uPA, respectively) demonstrating that the plasminogen activation plays an important role in follicular wall degradation during ovulation. Other animal models with female infertile phenotype were also described by Edelmann *et al.* 1996; Nakayama *et al.* 1996; Lee *et al* 1996; Sterneck *et al.* 1997; and Kumar *et al.* 1997.

Knockout mice not primarily affected on their female reproductive system but developing a final infertile phenotype have also been described. Female aromatase enzyme (ArKO) knockout mice demonstrated the consequences of a deficiency of aromatase activity in the formation of estrogens and therefore in the development of some organs; these mice displayed an underdeveloped external genitalia and uteri (Fisher *et al.* 1998). Ovarian hypofunction and hypoplastic uteri together with major organ dysfunction were described by Pietila *et al.* in 1997, while an infertile female phenotype was also observed in Zar1-null mice by Wu *et al.* in 2003, among others.

Knockout and Transgenic Mice Contribute to Elucidate the Molecular Mechanisms of Infertility

Ovarian follicle development is a very complex process which starts when the primordial germ cells (PGCs) reach the female gonad. At this stage PGCs, named *oogonia*, lose their motile characteristics and undergo multiple cell divisions. Some studies using transgenic mouse models have revealed that bone morphogenetic proteins (BMPs), such as BMP4 and BMP8, are involved in the establishment of PGCs (Lawson *et al.* 1999; Ying *et al* 2000, 2001). These cells interact with the type I activin receptor-like kinase (ALK) triggering signal transduction pathways resulting in gene expression pattern changes probably mediated by SMAD5 (Chang and Matzuk 2001; Chuva de Soussa Lopes *et al.* 2004). The cell interaction processes of PGCs are also very important for cell migration as revealed by PGCs lacking β1 integrin subunit (Anderson *et al.* 1999) being unable to interact with the extracellular matrix components (ECM) (García-Castro *et al.* 1997). Cell-cell communication between PGCs themselves or between PGCs and somatic cells via Cx43 gap junctional channels (Juneja *et al.* 1999) are essential for cell colonization as well as it is the interaction between the stromal cell-derived factor (SDF-1) with its receptor CXcr4 (Ara *et al.* 2003: Molyneaux *et al.* 2003).

At this point, oogonia cease dividing and enter meiosis to become oocytes. These cells are located in germ cell nests which after birth allow the formation of primordial follicles. The establishment of primordial follicle cells is the first step for follicle development although these follicles remain in resting stage until they receive signals to continue the folliculogenesis. An oocyte specific gene, the *factor in the germline α* (Figlα), has been shown to be essential for the formation of these primordial follicles by controlling the interactions between oocytes and the surrounding granulosa cells (Soyal *et al.* 2000). In addition, mice lacking nerve growth factor (NGF) display a reduce number of growing follicles in the ovary (Dissen *et al.* 2001) and alterations in its receptor, the *tyrosine kinase* (*Trk*), also affecting the follicle formation (Donovan *et al.* 1996; Spears *et al.* 2003). Animal models making use of genes coding for meiosis-specific proteins such as DMC1 or MSH5 provide also evidence that at least some meiotic genes play a very important role in meiotic chromosome synapses (Mandon-Pepin *et al.* 2002).

The process continues when the primordial follicles enlarge and become primary follicles in the presence of the zona pellucida surrounding the oocyte. Zona pellucida consists of ZP1, ZP2 and ZP3 glycoproteins which play a crucial role in folliculogenesis as shown in several animal models (Rankin *et al.* 1996, 1999, 2001) and it is confirmed in patients with fertilization failure undergoing IVF procedures and sharing genetic alterations in ZP proteins (Mannikko *et al.* 2005). An oocyte-specific factor, NOBOX, is also important for primary follicle formation as NOBOX-deficient mice show (Rajkovic *et al.* 2004). Similarly, some transcription factors of the Fork Head family have been shown to be essential for squamous to cuboidal granulosa cell transition, and therefore primary follicle formation, such as Foxl2 or Foxo3a (Schmidt *et al.* 2003; Castrillon *et al.* 2003; Batista *et al.* 2007).

Interestingly, Figlα and mutations in Foxl2, DMC1 or NOBOX have been related to premature ovarian failure (POF) in humans (Gersak *et al.* 2004; Pangas and Rajkovic *et al.* 2006; Mandon-Pepin *et al.* 2002) as well as NGF to the pathogenesis of PCOS in women (Bai *et al.* 2004).

Folliculogenesis continues with follicle granulosa cells then undergoing several divisions to form multiple layers and the primary follicles acquiring an outer layer of thecal cells becoming preantral follicles. All cells are communicated by gap junctional channels that allow small molecules to pass through. In this respect mice lacking the gap junction proteins Cx43 and Cx37 provide evidence that gap junctions are essential for follicular development into the preantral stage (Simon *et al.* 1997; Ackert *et al.* 2001). Gap junctions of Cx43 allow the intercellular communications between granulosa cells while gap junctions of Cx37 communicate granulosa cells with the oocyte. The blockage of folliculogenesis at preantral stage is also observed in transgenic mice deficient in γ-Glutamil transpeptidase GGT, enzyme responsible for converting glutathione (GSH) into cysteinil-glycine and γ-glutamic acid (Kumar *et al.* 2000).

At this point preantral follicles become antral follicles which are characterized by an antral cavity filled by follicular fluid. Most antral follicles will undergo atresia while the rest will continue their development process. Several pro-apoptotic and anti-apoptotic factors controlling atresia have shown to be important for the degradation of antral follicles, such as *Bcl2* or *Casps* (Ratts *et al.* 1995; Matikainen *et al.* 2001). The rest of antral follicles not affected by atresia grow to pre-ovulatory stage and ovulation takes place. In the further follicle remodelling, many inflammatory mediators are involved, for instance nitric oxide (Jablonka-Shariff and Olson 1998).

Reproductive defects affecting also the ovulation process are observed in female mice lacking prostaglandin E receptor (Ep2) (Hizaki *et al.* 1999); COX2, enzyme responsible for the synthesis of PGs (Matsumoto *et al.* 2001); inter-α-trypsin inhibitors (ITIs) (Suzuki et al. 2004); bikunin protein (Sato *et al.* 2001) or granulocyte macrophage colony-stimulating factor (GM-CSF) (Jasper *et al.* 2000); Gilchrist *et al.* 2000).

At the same time, during the process of oocyte maturation, the nucleus suffers modifications such as chromatin condensation, chromosome segregation and the extrusion of the first polar body. For resuming meiosis the phosphodiesterase 3A (PDE3A) via cAMP hydrolysis (Masciarelli *et al.* 2004); the Ercc1 (excision repair cross complementation group 1) (Hsia *et al.* 2003); the lunatic fringe gene (Hahn *et al.* 2005); the heat shock factors (Hsfs) (Christians *et al.* 2000); and some regulators of cell-cycle progression such as cyclin-dependent kinases (CDKs), Cyclin kinase (CK) and G protein coupled receptor 3 (GPR3) have all been shown to be important (Spruck *et al* 2003). For instance, $Cdk2^{-/-}$ and $Cdk4^{-/-}$ mice are also infertile (Ortega *et al.* 2003; Moons *et al.* 2002).

During folliculogenesis, oocyte companion cells also contribute to the follicular development by producing steroid hormones. As an example, the steroidogenic acute regulatory (STAR) protein promotes a very important step in the steroidogenesis pathway, in particular the transport of cholesterol inside mitochondria, as revealed in several studies (Caron *et al.* 1997; Hasegawa *et al.* 2000). In addition, the CYP19 (aromatase) knockout

(ArKO) model, already mentioned, lacks the capacity to produce estrogen (Fisher et al. 1998) and mice like these with alterations in the ability to respond to progesterone (Lydon *et al.* 1995) display also reproductive defects. In granulosa cells testosterone is aromatized to E_2, which in turn stimulate granulosa cell proliferation. Mice deficient in estrogen receptors confirm the very important role of E_2 (Lubahn *et al.* 1993, Krege *et al.* 1998, Dupon *et al.* 2000). Interestingly, patients with PCOS also display alterations of estrogen receptors such as ESr1 and ESR2 (Jakimiuk *et al.* 2002).

In addition, growth factors are also involved in regulating folliculogenesis. Oocytes express some members of TGFβ superfamily playing an essential role, such as Growth-differentiation factor 9 (GDF-9), BMP6 and BMP15; granulosa cells inhibins, activins,TGFβ1, TGFβ2 and TGFβ3; and theca cells BMP4 and BMP7 (Matzuk *et al.* 1992, 1995a, 1995b; Vassalli *et al* 1994; Dong *et al.* 1996; Guo *et al.* 1998; Cho *et al.* 2001; Yan *et al.* 2001; McMullen *et al.* 2002; Jorgez et al. 2004; Dixit *et al.* 2006).

The functional inactivation of GDF-9, a member of the TGFβ superfamily with the highest homology to BMP-15, has been shown to involve female infertility because of defects in folliculogenesis. Only primordial and primary one-layer follicles are observed in the periphery of the ovary of female GDF-9-deficient mice, and the oocyte degeneration occurs soon after formation of these follicles (Dong *et al.* 1996). In the absence of GDF-9 the follicles do not reach the secondary stage and are incompetent to recruit theca cells around the follicles. In addition, up-regulation of kit ligand and inhibin α is observed (Carabatsos *et al.* 1998; Elvin *et al.* 1999). The absence of GDF9 at the early follicle stage alters the differentiation program of the granulosa cells around. Thus, GDF-9 is essential for granulosa cell growth and differentiation and thecal layer formation, therefore regulating the somatic cell function.

Although activins do not appear to be essential for folliculogenesis, the absence of inhibins interferes with normal late stage folliculogenesis in mice (Matzuk *et al.* 1992; Vassalli *et al* 1994; Matzuk *et al.* 1995a, 1995 b). Female mice lacking FSHβ have an early block in folliculogenesis at the preantral stage (Kumar *et al.* 1997), while those lacking activin receptor type II (ActRII) have a later defect presenting a deficit of antral follicles and follicular atresia as well as rare corpora lutea. Consistent with the very important role of this receptor in the anterior pituitary, pituitary and serum levels of FSH were reduced (Matzuk *et al* 1995a).

TGFβ signalling pathways involve SMAD proteins and some of these molecules have also been described playing a critical role in folliculogenesis such as Smad3 (Zhu *et al.* 1998; Datto *et al.* 1999; Tomic et al. 2002, 2004). Granulosa cells also synthesize anti-Mullerian hormone (AMH) which inhibits the recruitment of primordial follicles and decreases the responsiveness of growing follicles to follicle stimulating hormone (FSH). Mice overexpressing *Amh* and AMHKO mice are infertile and have contributed to clarify the role played by AMH (Berhringer *et al.* 1990, 1994; Durlinger *et al.* 1999, 2001).

Together with autocrine and paracrine factors, endocrine regulatory elements play also and essential role in folliculogenesis, in particular in the late stages of this process. This is the case of FSH and LH hormones produced by the anterior pituitary. Mice lacking the ability to secrete or respond to FSH reveal that this hormone is necessary for follicular growth to the antral and pre-ovulatory stages (Kumar *et al.* 1997; Dierich *et al.* 1998; Abel *et al.* 200, 2003); and transgenic mice overexpressing FSH display increase steroid levels, produce ovarian cysts and cause infertility (Kumar *et al.* 1999). Mice with an ovarian phenotype unable to respond to LH hormone confirm that for the latest stages of follicular maturation and ovulation event, LH is absolutely necessary (Lei *et al.* 2001; Chudgar *et al.* 2005; Pakarainen *et al.* 2005a, 2005b) while mice that maintain chronically elevated LH levels show increased amounts of progesterone, testosterone and E_2 but also an infertile phenotype (Risma *et al.* 1995). In addition, Meehan *et al.* in 2005 reported a mouse model with a chronic LHR activation and a very early sex development.

On the other hand, cytokines have also been described critical to the success of the reproductive process, not only in a direct way but also in an indirect one, mediating immune tolerance and suppression. Conventionally, cytokines are soluble factors mediating cell signalling in the context of the immune system and group interleukins (ILs), tumor necrosis factor (TNF) and colony stimulating factors (GSFs). However, some growth factors as TGFs and endocrine hormones as the growth hormone (GH) are now considered also as cytokines and therefore, the function of cytokines seems to be not actually restricted to the immune system. For instance, it is well known that cytokines, such as IL-1β and TNF-α, participate in cell-cell signalling inside the ovary, in particular between the oocyte and its surrounding cells, and others, like INF-γ and GM-CSF, produced by resident macrophages in the ovary, promote oocyte development (see review in Wu *et al.* 2004; Knight and Glister 2006). Interestingly, female TGF-β1 knockout mice developed on an immunodeficient background display an impaired ovarian function (Ingman *et al.* 2006). Activins, closely related to TGF-βs, are also involved in the ovarian biology and at a later stage such as placental development and endometrial decidualization (Qu and Thomas 1995; Caniggia *et al.* 1997; Tierney and Giudice 2004). Female mice lacking colony-stimulating factor-1 (CSF-1) or granulocyte macrophage-CSF (GM-CSF), both of them cytokines, exhibit defects in reproductive function as well (Araki *et al.* 1996; Robertson *et al.* 1999, 2001; Jasper *et al.* 2000; Cohen *et al.* 2002).

As already mentioned, for embryo implantation to occur the expression of Leukaemia inhibitory factor (LIF) is mandatory, as it is revealed by the failure of blastocysts to attach to the endometrial epithelium in LIF knockout mice (Stewart *et al.* 1992), and even a more severe phenotype is obtained when the specific LIF receptor is knocked out (Ware *et al.* 1995).

In a recent paper, the analysis of transgenic mice over-expressing the transcription factor Foxj2 revealed a lethal effect involving developmental blockage and infertility (Martin et al. 2008) Abnormal embryos were rapidly reabsorbed within the decidual tissue. In the same paper, two target genes were described: the gene coding for the gap junctional protein Cx-43 and the gene coding for the cell adhesion molecule E-cadherin (E-Cad). It is well known that Cx43 plays a pivotal role in mouse follicular development, being the most widely expressed connexin in the human endometrium and is also known to be important in several pathological and physiological processes such as embryo implantation (Jahn *et al.* 1995; Granot *et al.* 2000; Gabriel *et al.* 2004; Tanmahasamut *et al.* 2005; Grümmer *et al.* 1996, 2004). On the other hand, E-Cad, a protein involved in cell adhesion events and in mediating the compaction process of mouse preimplantational embryos, is also important for the transition from compacted morulae to the formation of the blastocyst, thereby ensuring the correct establishment of adhesion junctions in the trophectoderm (Peyriéras *et al.* 1983; Larue *et al* 1994; Kan *et al.* 2007). It seems reasonable to ask ourselves whether irregularities at the transcriptional regulation level of Cx43 and E-Cad can compromise any of the following processes: oocyte maturation, early development, implantation process, and therefore female reproductive capability. The infertility phenotype observed for Foxj2 transgenic mice could be the natural consequence of a de-regulated expression of Cx43 and E-Cad at transcriptional level due to FoxJ2 over-expression (Martin *et al.* 2008).

More recently, SGOL2 (Shungoshin-2) has been described as an essential protein for protecting centromeric cohesion during meiosis; the disruption of the gene encoding mouse SGOL2 lead to the formation of aneuploid gametes that give rise to infertility (Llano *et al.* 2008). Additionally, MAPK3/1 (ERK1/2) (extracellular signal-regulated kinases 1 and 2) in ovarian granulosa cells have been reported to be absolutely necessary for LH-induced oocyte resumption of meiosis process, as well as ovulation and further luteinization (Fan *et al.* 2009).

Conclusion

In the last few years, several key transgenic and knockout mouse models have contributed to elucidate the mechanisms leading to follicle activation, dominance and survival, oocyte resumption of meiosis and growth/differentiation of the companion granulosa cells. Animal models have also helped defining the roles of extraovarian and intraovarian factors in ovarian functions as well as the biological processes involved in preimplantation/implantation and early embryo development.

All of these findings have enormously contributed to the understanding of the molecular basis of human reproduction resulting in tremendous advances in this area of biomedical research and improved treatment of female infertility. This progress is expected to continue in the coming years and we are confident that there will be more contributions from the gene knockout and transgenic mice field in the near future.

References

Abel, M. H., Huhtainiemi, I., Pakarinen, P., Kumar, T. R. and Charlton, H. M. (2003). Age-related uterine and ovarian hypertrophy in FSH receptor knockout ans FSHb subunit knockout mice. *Reproduction, 125*, 165-173.

Abel, M. H., Wootton, A. N., Wilkins, V., Huhtaniemi, I., Knight, P. G. and Charlton, H. M. (2000). The effect of a null mutation in the follicle-stimulating hormone receptor gene on mouse reproduction. *Endocrinology, 141*, 1795-1803.

Ackert, C. L., Gittens, J. E., O'Brien, M. J., Eppig, J. J. and Kidder, G. M. (2001). Intercellular communication via connexion43 gap junctions is required for ovarian folliculogenesis in the mouse. *Dev. Biol., 233*, 258-270.

Anderson, R., Fassler, R., Georges-Labouesse, E., Hynes, R. O., Bader, B. L., Kreidberg, J. A., Schaible, K., Heasman, J. and Wylie. (1999). Mouse primordial germ cells lacking β1 integrins enter the germline but fail to migrate normally to the gonads. *Development, 126*, 1655-1664.

Ara, T., Nakamura, Y., Egawa, T., Sugiyama, T., Abe, K., Kishimoto, T., Matsui, Y. and Nagasawa, T. (2003). Impaired colonization of the gonads by primordial germ cells in mice lacking a chemokine, stromal cell-derived factor-1 (SDF-1). *Proc. Natl. Acad. Sci.*, USA, *100*, 5319-5323.

Araki, M., Fukumatsu, Y., Katabuchi, H., Shultz, L. D., Takahashi, K. and Okamura, H. (1996). Follicular development and ovulation in macrophage colony-stimulating factor-deficient mice homozygous for the osteopetrosis (op) mutation. *Biol. Repro., 54*, 478-484.

Bai, Y. H., LIM, S. C., Song, C. H., Bae, C. S., Jin, C. S., Choi, B. C., Jang, C. H., Lee, S. H. and Pak, S. C. (2004). Electro-acupuncture reverses nerve growth factor abundance in experimental polycystic ovaries in the rat. *Gynecol. Obst. Invest., 57*, 80-85.

Batista, F., Vaiman, D., Dausset, J., Fellous, M. and Veitia, R. A. (2007). Potential target of FOXL2, a transcription factor involved in craniofacial and follicular development, identified by transcriptomics. *Proc. Natl. Acad. Sci.* USA., *104*, 3330-3335.

Behringer, R. R., Cate, R. L., Froelick, G. J., Palmiter, R. D. and Brinster, R. L. (1990). Abnormal sexual development in transgenic mice chronically expressing mullerian inhibiting substance. *Nature, 345*, 167-170.

Behringer, R. R., Finegold, M. J. and Cate, R. L. (1994). Mullerian-inhibiting substance function during mammalian sexual development. *Cell, 79*, 415-425.

Boivin, J., Bunting, L., Collins, J. A. and Nygren, K. G. (2007). International estimates of infertility prevalence and treatment-seeking: potential need and demand for infertility medical care. *Hum. Reprod., 22*, 1506-1512.

Caniggia, I., Lye, S. J. and Cross, J. C. (1997). Activin is a local regulator of human cytotrophoblast cell differentiation. *Endocrinology, 138*, 3976-3986.

Carabatsos, M. J., Elvin, J. A., Matzuk, M. M. and Albertini, D. F. (1998). Characterization of oocyte and follicle development in growth differentiation factor-9-deficient mice. *Dev. Biol., 203*, 373-384.

Caron, K. M., Soo, S. C., Wetsel, W. C., Stocco, D. M., Clark, B. J. and Parker, K. L. (1997). Targeted disruption of the mouse gene encoding steroidogenic acute regulatory protein provides insights into congenital lipoid adrenal hyperplasia. *Proc. Natl. Acad. Sci.*, USA, *94*, 11540-11545.

Castrillon, D. H., Miao, L., Kollipara, R., Horner, J. W. and Depinho, R. A. (2003). Suppression of ovarian follicle activation in mice by the transcription factor Foxo3a. *Science, 301*, 215-218.

Chang, H. and Matzuk, M. M. (2001). Smad 5 is required for mouse primordial germ cell development. *Mech. Dev., 104*, 61-67.

Cho, B. N., McMullen, M. L., Pei, L., Yates, C. J. and Mayo, K. E. (2001). Reproductive deficiencies in transgenic mice expressing the rat inhibina-subunit gene. *Endocrinology, 142*, 4994-54004.

Christians, E., Davis, A. A., Thomas, S. D. and Benjamin, I. J. (2000). Maternal effect of Hsf1 on reproductive success. *Nature, 407*, 693-694.

Chudgar, D., Lei, Z. and Rao, Ch.V. (2005). Orthotopic transplantation of LH receptor knockout and wildtype ovaries. *Life Sci., 77*, 2656-2662.

Chuva de Sousa Lopes, S. M., Roclen, B. A., Monteiro, R. M., Emmems, R., Lin, H. Y., Li, E., Lawson, K. A. and Mummery, C. L. (2004). Connective tissue growth factor expression and Smad signalling during mouse heart development and myocardial infarction. *Dev. Dyn., 231*, 542-550.

Cohen, P. E., Zhu, L., Nishimura, K. and Pollard, J. W. (2002). Colony-stimulating factor 1 regulation of neuroendocrine pathways that control gonadal function in mice. *Endocrinology, 143*, 1413-1422.

Colledge, W. H., Carlton, M. B., Udy, G. B. and Evans, M. J. (1994). Disruption of c-mos causes parthenogenetic development of infertilized mouse eggs. *Nature, 370*, 65-68.

Datto MB, Frederick JP, Pan L, Borton AJ, Zhuang Y, Wang XF. (1999). Targeted disruption of Smad3 reveals an essential role in transforming growth factor beta-mediated signal transduction. *Mol. Cell Biol., 19*, 2495-2504.

Di Giacomo, M., Barchi, M., Baudat, F., Edelmann, W., Keeney, S. and Jasin, M. (2005). Distinct DNA-damage-dependent and –independent responses drive the loss of oocytes in recombination-defective mouse mutants. *Proc. Natl. Acad. Sci.*, USA, *102*, 737-742.

Dierich, A., Sairam, M. R., Monaco, L., Fimia, G. M., Gansmuller, A., LeMeur, M. and Sassone–Cori, P. (1998). Impairing follicle-stimulating hormone (FSH) signalling in vivo: targeted disruption of the FSH receptor leads to aberrant gametogenesis and hormonal imbalance. *Proc. Natl. Acad. Sci., USA, 95*, 13612-13617.

Dissen, G. A., Romero, C., Hirshfield, A. N. and Ojeda, S. R. (2001). Nerve growth factor is required for early follicular development in the mammalian ovary. *Endocrinology, 142*, 2078-2086.

Dixit, H., Rao, L. K., Padmalatha, V. V., Kanakavalli, M., Deenadayal, M., Gupta, N., Chakrabarty, B. and Singh, L. (2006). Missense mutations in the BMP15 gene are associated with ovarian failure. *Hum. Gent., 119*, 408-415.

Dong, J., Albertini, D. F., Nishimori, K., Kumar, T. R., Lu, N. and Matzuk, M. M. (1996). Growth differentiation factor-9 is required during early ovarian folliculogenesis. *Nature, 383*, 531-535.

Dong, J., Albertini, D. F., Nishimori, K., Kumar, T. R., Lu, N. and Matzuk, M. M. (1996). Growth differentiation factor-9 is required during early ovarian folliculogenesis. *Nature, 383*, 531-535.

Donovan, M. J., Hahn, R., Tessarollo, L. and Hempstead (1996). Identification of an essential nonneuronal function of neurotrophin 3 in mammalian cardiac development. *Nat. Genet., 14*, 210-213.

Dupont, S., Krust, A., Gansmuller, A., Dierich, A., Chambon, P. and Mark, M. (2000). Effect of single and compound knockouts of estrogen receptors α (Erα) and β (ERβ) on mouse reproductive phenotypes. *Development, 127*, 4277-4291.

Durlinger, A. L., Grujters, M. J., Kramer, P., Karels, B., Kumar, T. R., Matzuk, M. M., Rose, U. M., de Jong, F. H., Uilenbroek, J. T., Grootegoed, J. A. et al. (2001). Anti-Mullerian hormones attenuates the effects on follicle development in the mouse ovary. *Endocrinology, 142*, 4891-4899.

Durlinger, A. L., Kramer, P., Karels, B., de Jong, F. H., Uilenbroek, J. T., Grootegoed, J. A. and Themmen, A. P. (1999). Control of primordial follicle recruitment by anti-Mullerian hormone in the mouse ovary. *Endocrinology, 140*, 5789-5796.

Edelmann, W., Cohen, P. E., Kane, M., Lau, K., Morrow, B., Bennett, S., Uman, A., Kunkel, T., Cattoretti, G., Chaganti, R., Pollard, J. W., Kolodner, RD. and Kuchelapati, R. (1996). Meiotic pachytene in MLH1-defcient mice. *Cell, 85(7)*, 1125-1134.

Elvin, J. A., Yan, C., Wang, P., Nishimori, K. and Matzuk, M. (1999). Molecular characterization of the follicle defects in the growth differentiation factor-9-deficinet ovary. *Mol. Endocrinol., 13*, 1018-1034.

Fan, H., Liu, Z., Shimada, M., Sterneck, E., Johnson, P. F., Hedrick, S. M. and Richards, J. S. (2009). MAPK3/1 (ERK1/2) in ovarian granulosa cells are essential for female fertility. *Science, 324*, 938-941.

Fisher, C. R., Graves, K. H., Parlow, A. F. and Simpson, E. R. (1998). Characterization of mice deficient in aromatase (ArKO) because of targeted disruption of the cyp19 gene. *Proc. Natl. Acad. Sci.,* USA., *95*, 6965-697.

Garcia-Castro, M. I., Anderson, R., Heasman, J. and Wylie. (1997). Interactions between germ cells and extracellular matrix glycoproteins during migration and gonad assembly in the mouse embryo. *J. Cell Biol., 138*, 471-480.

Gersak, K., Harris, S. E., Smale, W. J. and Shelling, A. N. (2004). A novel 30 bp deletion in the FOXL2 gene in a phenotypically normal woman with primary amenorrhoea: Case report. *Human Reprod., 19*, 2767-2770.

Gilchrist, R. B., Rove, D. B., Ritter, L. J., Robertson, S. A., Norman, R. J. and Armstrong, D. T. (2000). Effect of granulocyte-macrophage colony-stimulating factor deficiency on ovarian follicular cell function. *J. Reprod. Fertil., 120*, 283-292.

Guo, Q., Kumar, T. R., Woodruff, T., Hadsell, L. A., DeMayo, F. J. and Matzuk, M. M. (1998). Overexpression of mouse follistatin causes reproductive defects in transgenic mice. *Mol. Endocrinol., 12*, 96-106.

Hahn KL, Johson J, Beres BJ, Howard S, Wilson-Rawls. 2005. Lunatic fringe null female mice are infertile due to defects in meiotic maturation. *Development, 132*, 817-828.

Hizaki, H., Segi, E., Sugimoto, Y., Hirose, M., Saji, T., Ushikubi, F., Matsuoka, T., Noda, Y., Tanaka, T., Yoshida, N. et al. (1999). Abortive expansion of the cumulus and impaired infertility in mice lacking the prostaglandin E receptor subtype EP2. *Proc. Natl. Acad. Sci. USA, 96*, 10501-10506.

Hsia, K. T., Millar, M. R., King, S., Selfridge, J., Redhead, N. J., Melton, D. W. and Saunders, P. T. (2003). DNA repair gene Ercc 1 is essential for normal spermatogenesis and oogenesis and for functional integrity of germ cell DNA in the mouse. *Development, 130*, 369-378.

Ingman, W. V., Robker, R. L., Woittiez, K. and Robertson, S. A. (2006). Null mutation in transforming growth factor beta 1 disrupts ovarian function and causes oocyte incompetence and early embryo arrest. *Endocrinology, 147*, 835-845.

Jablonka-Shariff, A. and Olson, L. M. (1998). The role of nitric oxide in oocyte meiotic maturation and ovulation: meiotic abnormalities of endothelial nitric oxide synthase knock-out mouse oocytes. *Endocrinology, 139*, 2944-2954.

Jakimuik, A. J., Weitsman, S. R., Yen, H. W., Bogusiewicz, M. and Magoffin, D. A. (2002). Estrogen receptor alpha and beta expression in theca and granulose cells from women with polycystic ovary syndrome. *J. Clin. Endocrinol. Metab., 87*, 5532-5538.

Jasper, M. J., Robertson, S. A., Van der Hoek, K. H., Bonello, N., Brannstrom, M. and Norman, R. J. (2000). Characterization of ovarian function in granulocyte-macrophage colony-stimulating factor-deficient mice. *Biol. Reprod., 62*, 704-713.

Jorgez, C. J., Klysik, M., Jamin, S. P., Behrinh, R. R. and Matzuk, M. M. (2004). Granulosa cell-specific inactivation of follistatin causes female fertility defects. *Mol. Endocrinol., 18*, 953-967.

Juneja, S. C., Barr, K. J, Enders, G. C. and Kidder, G. M. (1999). Defects in the germ line and gonads of mice lacking connexin43. *Biol. Reprod., 60*, 1263-1270.

Knight, P. G. and Glister, C. (2006). TGF-beta superfamily members and ovarian follicle development. *Reproduction, 132*, 191-206.

Krege, J. H., Hodgin, J. B., Couse, J. F., Enmark, E., Warner, M., Mahler, J. F., Sar, M., Korach, K. S., Gustafsson, J. A. and Smithies, O. (1998). Generation and reproductive phenotypes of mice lacking estrogen receptor β. *Proc. Natl. Acad. Sci., USA, 95*, 15677-15682.

Kumar, T. R., Palapattu, G., Wang, P., Woodruff, T. K., Boime, I., Byrne, M. C. and Matzuk, M. M. (1999). Transgenic models to study gonadotropin function: the role of follicle-stimulating hormone in gonadal growth and tumorigenesis. *Mol. Endocrinol., 13*, 851-865.

Kumar, T. R., Wang, Y., Lu, N. and Matzuk, M. M. (1997). Follicle stimulating hormone is required for ovarian follicle maturation but not male fertility. *Nat. Genet., 15*, 201-204.

Kumar, T. R., Wiseman, A. L., Kala, G., Kala, S. V., Matzul, M. M. and Lieberman, M. W. (2000). Reproductive defects in γ-glutamyl transpeptidase-deficient mice. *Endocrinology, 141*, 4270-4277.

Lawson, K. A., Dunn, N. R., Roelen, B. A., Zeinstra, L. M., Davis, A. M., Wright, C. V., Korving, J. P. and Hogan, B. L. (1999). Bmp4 is required for the generation of primordial germ cells in the mouse embryo. *Genes Dev., 13*, 424-436.

Lee, S. L., Sadovsky, Y., Swirnoff, Polish, J. A., Goda, P., Gavrilina and Milbrandt, J. (1996). Luteinizing hormone deficiency and female infertility in mice lacking the transcription factor NGFI-A (Erg-1). *Science, 273*, 1219-1221.

Lei, Z. M., Mishra, S., Zou, W., Xu, B., Foltz, M., Li, X. and Rao, C. V. (2001). Targeted disruption of luteinizing hormone/human chorionic gonadotropin receptor gene. *Mol. Endocrinol., 15*, 184-200.

Leonardsson, G., Peng, X. R., Liu, K., Nordstrom, L., Carmeliet, P., Mulligan, R., Collen, D. and Ny, T. (1995). Ovulation efficiency is reduced in mice that lack plasminogen activator gene function: functional redundancy among physiological plasminogen activators. *Proc. Natl. Acad. Sci.,* USA., *92*, 12446-12450.

Llano, E., Gómez, R., Gutiérrez-Caballero, C., Herrán, Y., Sánchez-Martín, M., Vázquez-Quinones, L., Hernández, T., de Alava, E., Cuadrado, A., Barbero, J. L., Suja, J. A. and Pendás, A. M. (2008). Shugosin-2 is essential for the completion of meiosis but not for mitotic cell division in mice. *Genes Dev., 22*, 2400-2413.

Lubahn, D. B., Moyer, J. S., Golding, T. S., Couse, J. F., Korach, K. S. and Smithies, O. (1993). Alteration of reproductive function but not prenatal sexual development after insertion disruption of the mouse estrogen receptor gene. *Proc. Natl. Acad. Sci.,* USA., *90*, 11162-11166.

Lydon, J. P., DeMayo, F. J., Funk, C. R., Mani, S. K., Hughes, A. R., Montgomery, C. A. Jr., Shyamala, G., Conneely, O. M. and O'Malley, B. W. (1995). Mice lacking progesterone receptor exhibit pleiotropic reproductive abnormalities. *Genes Dev., 9*, 2266-2278.

Mandon-Pepin, B., Debois, C., Mastsuda, F., Cotinot, C., Wolgemuth, D. J., Smith, K., McElreavey, K., Nicolas, A. and Fellous, M. (2002). Human infertility: meiotic genes as potential candidates. *Gynecol. Obstet. Fertil., 10*, 817-821.

Mannikko, M., Tormala, R. M., Tuuri, T., Haltia, A., Martikainen, H., Ala-Kokko, L., Tapanainen, J. S. and Lakkakorpi, J. T. (2005). Association between sequence variations in genes encoding human pellucida glycoproteins and fertilization failure in IVF. *Human Reprod., 20(6)*, 1578-1585.

Martin-de-Lara, F., Sánchez-Aparicio, P., Arias de la Fuente, C. and Rey-Campos, J. (2008). Biological effects of FoxJ2 over-expression. *Transgenic Res., 17*, 1131-1141.

Masciarelli, S., Horner, K., Liu, C., Park, S. H., Hinckley, M., Hockman, S., Nedachi, T., Jin, C., Conti, M. and Manganiello, V. (2004). Cyclic nucleotide phospodiesterase 3A-deficient mice as a model of female infertility. *J. Clin. Invest., 114*, 196-205.

Matikainen, T., perez, G. I., Zheng, T. S., Kluzak, T. R., Rueda, B. R. Flavell, R. A. and Tilly, J. L. (2001). Caspase-3 gene knockout defines cell linage specificity for programmed cell death signalling in the ovary. *Endocrinology, 142*, 2468-2480.

Matsumoto, H., Ma, W., Smalley, W., Trzaskos, J., Breyer, R. M. and Dey, S. K. (2001). Diversification of cyclooxygenase-2-deived prostaglandins in ovulation and implantation. *Biol. Repro., 64*, 1557-1565.

Matzuk, M. M., Finegold, M. J., Su, J. G. J,, Hsueh, A. J. W. and Bradley, A. (1992). α-Inhibin is a tumor–suppressor gene with gonadal specificity in mice. *Nature, 360*, 313-319.

Matzuk, M. M., Kumar, T. R. and Bradley, A. (1995a). Different phenotype for mice deficient in either activins or activins receptor type II. *Nature, 374*, 356-360.

Matzuk, M. M., Kumar, T. R., Vassalli, Bickenbach, J. R., Roop, D. R., Jaenisch, R. and Bradley, A. (1995b). Functional analysis of activins in mammalian development. *Nature, 374*, 354-356.

McMullen, M. L., Cho, B. N., Yates, C. J. and Mayo, K. E. (2001). Gonadal pathologies in transgenic mice expressing the rat inhibin a-subunit. *Endocrinology, 142*, 5005-5014.

Meehan, T. P., Harmon, B. G., Overcast, M. E., Yu, K. K., Camper, S. A., Puett, D. and Narayan, P. (2005). Gonadal defects and hormonal alterations in transgenic mice expressing a single chain human chorionic gonadotropin–lutropin receptor complex. *J. Mol. Endocrinol., 34*, 489-503.

Molyneaux, K. A., Zinszner, H., Kunwar, P. S., Schaible, K., Stebler, J., Sunshine, M. J., O'Brien, W., Raz, E., Littman, D., Wylie, C. et al. (2003). The chemoline SDF1/CXCL12 and its receptor CXCR4 regulate mouse germ cell migration and survival. *Development, 130*, 4279-4286.

Moons, Y., Jirawatnotai, S., Tsutsui, T., Franks, R., Parlow, A. F., Hales, D. B., Gibori, G., Fazleabas, A. T. and Kiyokawa, H. (2002). Intact follicular maturation and defective luteal function in mice deficient for cyclin-dependent kinase-4. *Endocrinology, 143*, 647-654.

Nakayama, K., Ishida, N., Shirane, M., Inomata, A., Inoue, T., Shishido, N., Horli, I., Loh, D. Y. and Nakayama, K. (1996). Mice lacking p27(kip1) display increased body size, multiple organ hyperplasia, retinal dysplasia, and pituitary tumors. *Cell, 85*, 707-720.

Ortega, S., Prieto, I., Odakima, J., Martin, A., Dubus, P., Sotillo, R., Barbero, J. L., Malumbres, M. and Barbacid, M. (2003). Cyclin-dependent kinase 2 is essential for meiosis but not for mitotic cell division in mice. *Nat. Genet., 35*, 25-31.

Ottolenghi, C., Omari, S., García-Ortiz, J. E., Uda, M., Crisponi, L., Forabosco, A., Pilia, G. and Schlessinger (2005). Foxl2 is required for commitment to ovary differentiation. *Human Mol. Genet., 15*, 2053-2062.

Pakarainen, T., Zhang, F. P., Nurmi, L., Poutanen, M. and Huhtaniemi, I. (2005a). Knockout of luteinizing hormone receptor abolished the effects of follicle-stimulating hormone on preovulatory maturation and ovulation of mouse graafian follicles. *Mol. Endocrinol., 19*, 2591-2602.

Pakarainen, T., Zhang, F. P., Poutanen, M. and Huhtaniemi, I. (2005b). Fertility in luteinizing hormone receptor knockout mice after wild-type ovary transplantation demonstrates redundancy of extragonadal luteinizing hormone action. *J. Clin. Invest., 115*, 1862-1868.

Pangas, S. A. and Rajkovic, A. (2006). Transcriptional regulation of early oogenesis: in search of masters. *Hum. Repro. Update, 12*, 65-76.

Pietila, M., Alhonen, L., Halmekyto, M., Kanter, P., Janne, J. and Porter, C. W. (1997). Activation of polyamine catabolism profoundly alters tissue polyamine pools and affects hair growth and female fertility in transgenic mice overexpressing spermidinespermine N^1-Acetyltransferase. *J. Biol. Chem., 272*, 18746-18751.

Qu, J. and Thomas, K. (1995). Inhibin and activin production in human placenta. *Endocr. Rev., 16*, 485-507.

Rajkovic, A., Panga, S. A., Ballow, D., Suzumori, N. and Matzuk, M. M. (2004). NOBOX deficiency disrupts early folliculogenesis and oocyte-specific gene expression. *Science, 305*, 1157-1159.

Rankin, T., Familari, m., Lee, E., Ginsberg, A., Dwyer, N., Blanchette-Mackie, J., Drago, J., Westphal, H. and Dean, J. (1996). Mice homozygous for an insertional mutation in the zp3 gene lack a zona pellucida and are infertile. *Develpemnt, 122*, 2903-2910.

Rankin, T., Talbot, P., Lee, E. and Dean, J. (1999). Abnormal zonae pellucidae in mice lacking ZP1 result in early embryonic loss. *Development, 126*, 3847-3855.

Rankin, T. L., O'Brien, M., Lee, E., Wigglesworth, K., Eppig, J. and Dean, J. (2001). Defective zonae pellucidae in Zp2-null mice disrupt folliculogenesis, fertility and development. *Development, 128*, 1119-1126.

Ratts, V. S., Flaws, J. A., Kolp, R., Sorenson, C. M. and Tilly, J. L. (1995). Ablation of bcl-2 gene expression decreases the numbers of oocytes and primordial follicles established in the post-natal female mouse gonad. *Endocrinology, 136*, 3665-3668.

Risma, K. A., Clay, C. M., Nett, T. M., Wagner, T., Yun, J. and Nilson, J. H. (1995). Targeted overexpression of luteinizing hormone in transgenic mice leads to infertility, polycystic ovaries, and ovarian tumors. *Proc. Natl. Acad. Sci.,* USA., *92*, 1322-1326.

Robertsons, S. A., Roberts, C. T., Farr, K. L., Dunn, A. R. and Seamark, R. F. (1999). Fertility impairment in granulocyte-macrophage colony-stimulating factor-deficint mice. *Biol. Reprod., 60*, 251-261.

Robertsons, S. A., Sjoblom, C., Jasper, M. J., Norman, R. J. and Seamark, R. F. (2001). Granulocyte-macrophage colony-stimulating factor promotes glucose transport and blastomere viability in murine preimplantation embryos. *Biol. Repro., 64*, 1206-1215.

Sato, H., Kajiwara, S., Kuroda, S., Horisawa, Y., Nakamura, N., Kaga, N., Nakinuma, C., Kato, K., Morishita, H., Niwa, et al. (2001). Impaired fertility in female mice lacking urinary trypsin inhibitor. *Biochem. Biophys. Res. Commun., 281*, 1154-1160.

Schmidt, D., Ovitt, C. E., Anlag, K., Fehsenfeld, S.., Gredsted, L., Treier, A. C. and Treier, M. (2003). The murine winged-helix transcription factor Foxl2 is required for granulosa cell differentiation and ovary maintenance. *Development, 131*, 933-942.

Simon, A. M., Goodenough, D. A., Li, E. and Paul, D. L. (1997). Female infertility in mice lacking connexin 37. *Nature, 385*, 525-9.

Soyal, S. M., Amleh, A. and Dean, J. (2000). FIGα, a germ cell-specific transcription factor required for ovarian follicle formation. *Development, 127*, 4645-4654.

Spears, N., Molinek, M. D., Robinson, L. L., Fulton, N., Cameron, H., Shimoda, K., Telfer, E. E., Anderson, R. A. and Price, D. J. (2003). The role of neurotrophin receptors in female germ-cell survival in mouse and human. *Development, 130*, 5481-5491.

Spruck, C. H., De Miguel, M. P., Smith, A. P., Ryan, A., Stein, P., Schultz, R. M., Lincoln, A. J., Donovan, P. J. and Reed, S. I. (2003). Requirements of Cks2 for the first metaphase/anaphase transition of mammalian meiosis. *Science, 300*, 647-650.

Sterneck, E., Tessarollo, L. and Johnson, P. F. (1997). An essential role for C/EBPbeta in female reproduction. *Genes Dev., 11*, 2153-2162.

Stewart, C. L., Kaspar, P., Brunet, L. J., Bhatt, H., Gadi, I., Kontgen, F. and Abbondanzo, S. J. (1992). Blastocyst implantation depends on maternal expression of leukaemia inhibitory factor. *Nature, 359*, 76-79.

Suzuki, M., Kobayashi, H., Tanaka, Y., Kanayama, N. and Terao, T. (2004). Reproductive failure in mice lacking inter-alpha-trypsin inhibitor (ITI)-ITI target genes in mouse ovary identified by microarray analysis. *J. Endocrinol., 183*, 29-38.

Tierney, E. P. and Giudice, L. C. (2004). Role of activin A as a mediator of in vitro endometrial stromal cell decidualization via the cyclic adenosine monophosphate pathway. *Fert. Steril., 81*, 899-903.

Tomic, D., Brodie, S. G., Deng, C., Hickey, J. K., Malkas, L. H. and Flaws, J. A. (2002). Samd3 may regulate follicular growth in the mouse ovary. *Biol. Reprod., 66*, 917-923.

Tomic, D., Miller, K. P., Kenny, H. A., Woodruff, T. K., Hoyer, P. and Flaws, J. A. (2004). Ovarian follicle development requires Smad3. *Mol. Endocrinol., 18*, 2224-2240.

Vassalli, A., Matzuk, M. M., Gardner, H. A. R,. Lee, K. F. and Jaenisch, R. (1994). Activin/inhibins βB subunit disruption leads to defects in eyelid development and female reproduction. *Gene Dev., 8*, 414-427.

Ware, C. B., Horowitz, M. C., Renshaw, B. R., Hunt, J. S., Liggitt, D., Koblar, S. A., Gliniak, B. C., McKenna, H. J., Papayannopoulou, T., Thoma, B., et al. (1995). Targeted disruption of the low-affinity leukaemia inhibitory factor recptor geen cuses placental, skeletal, neural and metabolic defects and results in perinatal death. *Development, 121*, 1283-1299.

Wu, R., Van der Hoek, K. H., Ryan, N. K., Norman, R. J. and Robker, R. L. (2004). Macrophage contributions to ovarian function. *Human Reprod. Update, 10*, 119-133.

Wu, X., Viveiros, M., Eppig, J., Bai, Y., Fitzpatrick, S. L. and Matzuk, M. M. (2003). Zygote arrest 1 (Zar1) is a novel maternal-effect gene critical for the oocyte-to-embryo transition. *Nature Genet., 33*, 187-191.

Yamada, Y. and Coffman, C. R. (2005). DNA damage-induced programmed cell death. Potential roles in germ cell development. *Ann. NY Acad. Sci., 1049*, 9-16.

Yan, C., Wang, P., DeMayo, J., DeMayo, F. J., Elvin, J. A., Carino, C., Prasad, S. V., Skinner, S. S., Dunbar, B. S., Dube, J. L., et al. (2001). Synergistic roles of bone morphogentic protein 15 and growth differentiation factor 9 in ovarian function. *Mol. Endocrinol., 15*, 854-866.

Ying, Y. and Zhao, G. Q. (2001). Cooperation of endoderm-derived BMP2 and extraembryonic ectoderm-derived BMP4 in primordial germ cell generation in the mouse. *Dev. Biol., 232*, 484-492.

Ying, Y., Liu, X. M., Marble, A., Lawson, K. A. and Zhao, G. Q. (2000). Requirement of Bmp8b for the generation of primordial germ cells in the mouse. *Mol. Endocrinol., 14*, 1053-1063.

Zhu, Y., Richardson, J. A., Parada, L. F. and Graff, J. M. (1998). Smad3 mutant mice develop metasatic colorectal cancer. *Cell, 94*, 703-714.

In: Infertility
Editors: R. Nascimento and H. V. Boas
ISBN: 978-1-62257-909-9

Chapter 7

Treatment of Endometriosis Associated with Infertility and Chronic Pelvic Pain

Julio Cesar Rosa e Silva, Juliana Meola, Ana Carolina Japur de Sá Rosa e Silva, Omero Benedicto Poli Neto, Francisco José Candido dos Reis and Antonio Alberto Nogueira
Department of Gynecology and Obstetrics, School of Medicine of Ribeirão Preto, University of São Paulo, Brazil

Abstract

Despite the significant heterogeneity in the clinical manifestations of endometriosis, a high prevalence of the disease is observed in infertile women, and in women with chronic pelvic pain. The socioeconomic impact of this enigmatic condition is high, and the data regarding the efficacy of the different therapeutic approaches is quite conflicting. Thus, the objective of this article is to describe the scientific evidence available regarding therapeutic modalities, and to provide recommendations for the treatment of infertility and chronic pelvic pain related to endometriosis. In patients with mild endometriosis, the suppression of ovarian function does not improve fertility, but the ablation of the lesions associated with adhesiolysis does seem to be more effective in improving fertility than the exclusive use of diagnostic laparoscopy.

There is insufficient evidence to determine whether surgical excision improves pregnancy rates in cases of moderate or severe endometriosis. In vitro fertilization (IVF) seems to be an adequate approach, especially in cases that involve other infertility factors and/or the failure of other treatments.

The use of GnRH for 3 to 6 months before IVF is recommended. With regard to pain relief, the suppression of ovarian function for 3 to 6 months in patients, whose endometriosis is laparoscopically confirmed, has been shown to reduce the pain associated with endometriosis. All of the medications studied seem to have similar efficacy, varying only in terms of adverse effects and cost. The ablation of endometriotic lesions reduces the pain associated with endometriosis, but is less effective in less severe cases of the disease.

The excision of endometriomas > 4 cm in diameter seems to improve the rate of natural fecundity, as well as the fertility rate obtained with assisted reproduction procedures. These procedures also reduce the levels of pain and the risk of recurrence. Finally, it is important to emphasize that there are countless controversies regarding the treatment of this disease, and that the recommendations described above should be revised as randomized controlled clinical trials with adequate patient enrollment generate evidence that is more reliable.

Keywords: Endometriosis, Treatment, Infertility, Chronic Pelvic Pain, Endometrioma, Assisted Reproduction

Introduction

Endometriosis is a disease that affects women of reproductive age and is characterized by the implantation and growth of endometrial tissue (glands and/or stroma) outside the uterine cavity. It has been observed in 5% to 10% of patients that have undergone gynecological laparotomies, 20% to 50% of infertile women [1], and 60% to 70% of patients with chronic pelvic pain [2].

This affliction can present with a wide variety of clinical manifestations. It is possible to find oligo or asymptomatic patients, patients with severe pelvic pain, patients with symptoms resulting from lesions in non-reproductive organs, and infertility. The symptoms associated with this disease have repercussions in all aspects of the patient's life, and one should pay special attention to all of the patient's complaints [3].

Treatment should always take into account the symptoms of the individual patient, and the impact the disease and its treatment has had on their quality of life. A specialized multi-disciplinary team should be, whenever possible, involved in an attempt to provide treatment capable of addressing all of the patient's biological, psychological, and social needs. In a didactic manner, we will subdivide the present article into sections concerning the treatment of infertility and the treatment of the chronic pelvic pain associated with endometriosis.

We will also present a systematic review of the most important and controversial topics in the literature regarding the treatment of the symptoms associated with this disease, while attempting to analyze the available data in a critical way, so as to highlight the evidence.

However, it is worth emphasizing that the vast majority of the available data, which provides evidence to support current treatments, is conflicting and will likely be revised as well-designed, prospective, randomized and controlled studies with larger patient populations are carried out. Such studies are likely to generate evidence that is more reliable.

1. Treatment of Infertility Associated with Endometriosis

1.1. Endometriosis and Fertility

In normal couples, fecundity varies from 0.15 to 0.20 per month and declines with age [4]. The monthly fecundity of infertile women with endometriosis is significantly lower and varies from 0.02 to 0.1 [5]. Some studies report that 20% to 50% of infertile women have endometriosis, and that 30% to 50% of the women with endometriosis are infertile, which suggests a possible role for endometriosis in the etiopathogenesis of infertility.

In cases of moderate and severe endometriosis, those in which morphologic involvement of the pelvic anatomy is generally identified, the association between this affliction and subsequent infertility is clear, although a clear demonstration of a causal relationship has not been established. In more mild cases of the disease, where mechanical changes in the reproductive tract are not observed, this association becomes even more tenuous. However, some studies have shown evidence of lower fecundity rates in this group of patients (from 0.019 to 0.024), when compared to normal fertile women (from 0.15 to 0.20) [6,7].

1.2. Clinical Medicinal Treatment

Several randomized and controlled clinical studies have demonstrated that the administration of danazol, progestins, or GnRH agonists are not effective for the treatment of infertility associated with mild cases of endometriosis. Thus, suppressing ovarian function, by means of hormone therapy, with the intention of improving fertility in cases of mild endometriosis is not effective, delays the possibility of pregnancy, and should not be offered as the only therapeutic approach [8].

There is no evidence that the transitory suppression of ovarian function subsequently improves fecundity in cases of moderate or severe endometriosis. As a result, we do not recommend this practice as an isolated therapy in clinical practice, and particularly not as a first line treatment. However, some studies suggest that there are increased gestation rates when prolonged ovarian suppression is coupled with the use of a GnRH agonist before the assisted reproductive cycle (AR). There are at least two case-controlled studies and one randomized controlled clinical trial (RCT) that support this approach [9-11]. The RCT in question evaluated 51 women in all stages of the disease that had received three months of treatment with GnRH analogs, and compared them with a group that did not receive any treatment before the AR cycle. The clinical pregnancy rate in the initiated cycle was 80% in the treated group versus 54% in the control group, and there was no difference in the gonadotrophin dosage used [11]. The principal critique of this study was that the reported pregnancy rate was much greater than the national average (33%) for the same year (as reported by the ASRM, the Society for Assisted Reproductive Technology).

One recent review by Cochrane suggests that the administration of GnRH analogs to women with endometriosis for a period of 3 to 6 months before in vitro fertilization (IVF) or intracytoplasmic sperm injection (ICSI) increases the likelihood of clinical pregnancy four fold [12]. Data concerning the potential adverse effects of this therapeutic approach on the mother or the fetus are not presently available. However, it is important to point out that in addition to the small sample size in this review (165 women), data on the severity of the disease, the presence and duration of infertility, the indication of the AR procedure, and age of the patients were not separately evaluated. Thus, the adoption of this practice should occur on an individualized basis and be discussed with patients, while taking into consideration other factors, such as other potential determinants of the success of the assisted reproductive procedures.

1.3. Surgical Treatment

The principal objectives of surgery in patients with endometriosis are to remove the largest amount of tissue possible and to reestablish the normal anatomy of the pelvis. Delicate handling of tissue and meticulous hemostasis are fundamental in preventing the formation of new adherences and endometrial foci [13].

The ablation of endometrial lesions associated with adhesiolysis in order to improve fertility in cases of mild endometriosis is effective when compared with diagnostic laparoscopy alone [14]. This statement is based on a systematic review and meta-analysis of two similar, although contradictory, randomized controlled clinical trials that examined the effectiveness of laparoscopic surgical ablation (plus adhesiolysis) relative to diagnostic laparoscopy alone, with regard to improved fecundity in patients with mild endometriosis. However, the evidence from the two available studies can be questioned. In an Italian study [7], where improved fecundity was not observed in the surgically treated group, the number of patients included was very small (101 patients). A Canadian study [6], which involved a larger patient population (341 women), showed a significantly higher monthly fecundity rate in the treated group when compared to the control group. However, we cannot determine if the patients knew whether they underwent surgical treatment during the laparoscopy or not, which introduces another bias in the data obtained. We have found no evidence that demonstrates the ablation method used, either electrosurgery, or laser, affects the fecundity rate after surgical treatment [6].

As a result, we suggest that until further studies are published, if the presence of mild endometriosis is identified during the performance of diagnostic laparoscopy on an infertile patient, one should carry out the surgical ablation of the lesions and adhesiolysis. The post surgical treatment, whether an assisted reproduction procedure or observation, should take into consideration other factors, such as the age of the patient, the duration of infertility, the type and results of previous treatments, and the presence or absence of an associated masculine factor, among others. On the other hand, the indication for a laparoscopic surgical approach is very questionable if the objective of the surgical ablation of the lesions and adhesiolysis is to improve fecundity in patients with a previous diagnosis of mild endometriosis. We believe that this practice should be individualized and discussed with the patient only in situations where, after a global examination of the case, the expected treatment seems likely to increase the possibility of spontaneous conception.

As for cases of moderate or severe endometriosis, only observational studies that have evaluated the influence of surgical treatment on gestation rates are available. Some studies [15-17] suggest that there is a negative correlation between the endometriotic stage and the cumulative rate of spontaneous pregnancy after the surgical removal of the endometrial lesions. However, this result was only found to be statistically significant in one study [17]. It is important to mention that data from different studies cannot be easily compared, since the completed surgical procedures, the extent of the surgeries, the ability of the surgeons, and other variables that determine the outcomes, certainly were not standardized [18].

To date, there are no controlled randomized clinical studies or meta-analyses that have evaluated whether the surgical removal of lesions in moderate or severe endometriosis improves gestation rates.

Thus, it is not possible to determine whether the surgical treatment of moderate or severe endometriosis improves subsequent rates of pregnancy, and the indication of this approach should be individualized. Among others factors, the evaluation of the indication for surgery should consider the age of the patient and the presence of other causes of infertility. Although controversial, we do not recommend postponing indicated AR procedures in infertile patients over 35 years of age in favor of surgical endometriosis management, given the reduction in reproductive potential inherent in further advancement of age.

1.4. Endometriomas

One recent review from Cochrane, whose objective was to determine the most effective surgical technique for the treatment of endometriomas, ablation or excision of the capsule, evaluated two randomized studies concerning the laparoscopic management of endometriomas larger than 3 cm [19]. Two RCT were included in the analysis.

The results demonstrated that laparoscopic excision of the capsule was associated with a reduction in the rate of endometrioma recurrence (OR: 0.41, CI 0.18-0.93), and with a reduction in the need for reintervention (OR 0.21, CI 0.05-0.79), as well as an increase in the rate of spontaneous pregnancy (evaluated from 12 to 24 months after the surgical intervention) in women with documented subfertility (OR 5.21, CI 2.04-13.29) [19]. Independent of the surgical technique utilized, it is recommended that part of the endometrioma's capsule be sent for anatomical-pathological analysis to confirm the clinical diagnosis, and to exclude the presence of a malignancy (estimated risk of a malignancy 0.7%) [19].

According to the latest publication by the European Society of Human Reproduction and Embryology, ESHRE [18], the laparoscopic excision of endometriomas > 4 cm in diameter improves fertility, as characterized by an increase in the rates of spontaneous gestation after surgical intervention when compared to draining and coagulation of the pseudocapsule [20,21]. Laparoscopic excision is at the same time associated with a decreased risk of cyst recurrence [22].

However, we believe that the adoption of surgical treatment as the exclusive approach for infertility associated with endometriosis should be considered on a case-by-case basis, as mentioned previously.

In cases where the use of assisted reproduction procedures is indicated, there remains some controversy as to the influence of the endometrioma on the results. Some studies report that the presence of endometrioma does not affect the results of IVF cycles. Others report a reduction in the response to the induction of ovulation, and in the number of embryos to be transferred, as well as increased spontaneous abortion rates. Although controversial and without concrete evidence, the latest publication by ESHRE [18] recommends the laparoscopic excision of endometriomas > 4 cm in diameter at the beginning of controlled ovarian stimulation, in order to obtain material for an anatomic-pathological diagnosis, to reduce the risk of infection, to facilitate technical access to the follicles during oocyte retrieval, and possibly, to improve ovarian response to the administration of endogenous gonadotrophins. However, this decision should be made on an individualized basis, and reconsidered with patients who have undergone prior surgical interventions.

On one hand, the evidence suggests there is a benefit from the excision of the endometrioma pseudocapsule in terms of reduced rates of recurrence and the reduced likelihood that reintervention will be necessary, as well as an increase in the rate of spontaneous pregnancy in subsequent months. On the other hand, a potential negative effect of this procedure is reduced ovarian follicular reserve [23-27].

However, other studies are necessary to clarify whether this damage is related to the surgical procedure or to the previous presence of the cyst [28]. In any event, this fact should be taken into consideration before and during the intraoperative, in order to determine the best surgical approach and to minimize the damage to apparently normal ovarian parenchyma.

1.5. Pre- and Post-Operative Treatment

There are no controlled randomized clinical trials (RCT) that evaluate the effect of hormonal treatment before surgical intervention.

Treatment with danazol or a GnRH agonist after surgery does not improve fertility when compared to the standard treatment [29-31]. Thus, in cases where the standard treatment is chosen for post-operative care, we do not recommend the routine use of hormone therapy to improve natural fecundity.

However, as previously described, the administration of GnRH analogs for a period of 3 to 6 months before in vitro fertilization (IVF) or intracytoplamic sperm injections (ICSI) in women with endometriosis increases the likelihood of clinical pregnancy by four fold [12]. Thus, in cases where the use of AR is indicated, this post-operative treatment can be adopted, but this decision should be made on an individualized basis and discussed with the patient, while taking into consideration the adverse effects of the use of GnRH analogs, the possible consequences of delaying the completion of the procedure, as well as other factors that may influence the success of the assisted reproduction procedures.

1.6. Assisted Reproduction Technologies

The controlled ovarian stimulation using clomiphene citrate or gonadotropins, along with intrauterine insemination, improves fertility in patients with mild endometriosis. We suggest that this practice can be adopted, while taking into consideration the age of the patient (preferentially younger than 35 years), the exclusion of a severe masculine factor, and the failure of previous similar attempts, noting the expected fecundity rates per cycle of from 0.095 to 0.129 [32,33].

There are no large controlled randomized clinical trials available that have definitively demonstrated the greater effectiveness of in vitro fertilization and embryo transfer (IVF-ET) relative to other methods for the treatment of infertility associated with endometriosis.

However, IVF-ET has been routinely offered to these patients, and according to the latest ESHERE guideline, it is an appropriate approach, especially in cases of tubal dysfunction, the presence of an associated male factor, and/or after the failure of other therapeutic measures [18]. Other factors, such as advanced age, the presence of a reduced ovarian follicular reserve, and the duration of infertility also should be considered when determining the treatment to be offered.

The possibly deleterious role of endometriosis on the results of IVF-ET procedures is controversial. A meta-analysis published in 2002 showed some evidence for lower pregnancy rates in patients undergoing IVF-ET with endometriosis, when compared to patients with tubular infertility [34]. However, this meta-analysis included older studies, which used laparoscopic oocyte retrieval and less effective protocols for ovarian stimulation. Indeed, some large databases, such as that from the Society for Assisted Reproductive Technology, have not observed an adverse effect from endometriosis on gestation rates after IVF-ET.

As previously mentioned, a recent review by Cochrane suggests that the administration of GnRH analogs for a period of 3 to 6 months before in vitro fertilization (IVF) or intracytoplasmic sperm injection (ICSI) in women with endometriosis increases the likelihood of clinical pregnancy by four fold [12]. However, the heterogeneity of the studies analyzed in this review make that conclusions questionable. Thus, this practice should be adopted on an individualized basis and discussed with the patient, while taking into consideration other factors that may influence the success of the assisted reproduction procedures.

2. Treatment of Endometriosis Associated with Pelvic Pain

2.1. Clinical Treatment of Endometriosis Associated with Pelvic Pain

The efficacy of the medications used for the treatment of endometriosis is based on the fact that endometriosis is responsive to hormones. Two physiological conditions, pregnancy and menopause, are frequently associated with the resolution of the pain caused by endometriosis. The pharmacological analogs of these conditions are progestogens and combined oral contraceptives, which lead to hormonal conditions similar to those seen during pregnancy, while the androgens and GnRH agonists (GNRHa) promote the suppression of endogenous estrogen production.

In light of the following documented evidence, we can conclude that the treatment of pelvic pain associated with endometriosis using medications is highly effective, with success rates ranging from 80% to 100% for improvement and symptom free intervals that can be as long as two years. The hormonal drugs investigated - medroxyprogesterone acetate, gestrinone, COC, danazol, and GnRH agonists are equally effective in pain relief. However, the adverse effects and the costs are different in each case, and should be taken into consideration when selecting a therapy [18].

2.1.1. Progestogens and Combined Oral Contraceptives

Although progesterone causes secretory changes to the endometrium during the luteal phase of the normal menstrual cycle, synthetic progestogens cause endometrial atrophy by reducing the synthesis of estrogen receptors. In 1958, Kirstner was the first to use this class of medication to treat endometriosis. He used high doses of progestogens, which lead to a state of pseudo-pregnancy [35].

Medroxyprogesterone acetate (MPA) is one of the most commonly used progestogens for the treatment of pelvic pain associated with endometriosis. However, the data from the literature on the subject is controversial. Luciano et al. showed improvements of 88% and 83% in dysmenorrhea and dispareunia, respectively, with a 50 mg/day oral dose of MPA [36]. The endometriosial cysts showed signs of atrophy and pseudo-decidualization in a biopsy performed during a later diagnostic laparoscopy [36]. However, in 2000 Harrison and Barry-Kinsella showed in a prospective, randomized, and placebo controlled study that this medication did not show a significantly greater improvement than placebo in controlling dysmenorrhea in patients with endometriosis after 12 weeks of continuous oral use at a dose of 50 mg/day [37]. In addition to a lack of efficacy, these patients presented with a high incidence of side effects (40%), such as acne, localized pain, and vasodilation, which was not better described in another similar study [37].

MPA is a contraceptive formulation that has been adopted by some researchers for the treatment of endometriosis. In one comparative controlled study that compared a 150 mg/day dose of MPA and a combined oral contraceptive, danazol, at a dose of 50 mg/day, the authors showed that the two treatments were equally and highly effective for the control of pain, especially after six months of treatment, and with patients reaching maximum satisfaction after twelve months. However, the use of MPA lead to high incidence of side effects, which were present in about 30% of the patients, but there was no evaluation of the effectiveness of this approach after twelve months of treatment [38].

Gestrinone, a progestogen with androgenic activity, has also been used to treat endometriosis and compared with GnRHa. Gestrinone seems to have a similar efficacy in controlling pain and providing patient satisfaction as GnRHa [39,40]. However, this medication has side effects that patients often do not wish to endure, such as amenorrhea, spotting, acne, hirsutism, edema, and weight gain that can reach 3 kilos after six months of treatment. The adequate dosage is between 200 and 300 mg/week, and patients should always be monitored for amenorrhea.

Other oral progestogens, such as cyproterone acetate, desogestrel, norethindrone acetate, levonorgestrel, and dydrogesterone, among others can be used, and have already been tested for the treatment of endometriosis, but more studies must be conducted to define their usefulness in patients with pelvic pain and endometriosis [41,42].

Other means of progestogen administration have been tested, such as subdermal implantation of etonorgestrel and the intrauterine slow release of levonorgestrel, the former with at least one pilot study in the literature showing good response and patient satisfaction [43]. There are some studies in the literature that demonstrate good effectiveness for the intrauterine system using levonorgestrel (IUS-LNG) for the relief of pain associated with endometriosis. In 1999, Vercellini et al., and then in 2001 Fedele et al. were the first to test IUS-LNG for the treatment of endometriosis, and showed it to be effective in controlling pain [44,45]. In 2005, Petta et al. published a prospective randomized controlled study showing an important reduction in secondary chronic pelvic pain and endometriosis in as early as the first month of use [46]. Associated with this clinical improvement, they also found a reduction in CA-125 serum levels, a tumor marker used in clinical practice to monitor endometriosis [47].

Although the data cited is promising, the patient population evaluated was small, and does not provide enough evidence to allow advocation of its routine use.

Combined oral contraceptives (COC) are the first choice for clinical treatment in many centers. In 1993, Vercellini et al. completed the first controlled study using this therapy comparing it with the use of GnRHa, and demonstrated that the use of COC, even when used cyclically (that is 21 days of hormone and 7 days without medication), had an effect similar to the administration of GnRHa in reducing pelvic pain associated with endometriosis [48]. There are still controversies associated with this therapy. Some studies have not demonstrated COC's post-operative effectiveness in postponing the timing of disease recurrence [49]. However, because this treatment is simple, inexpensive, easily taken, and shows good results in the literature, COC have been widely used to control pelvic pain associated with endometriosis. Despite its common use, the mechanism by which this treatment regimen acts on the foci of endometriosis is still not clear.

It is interesting to note that in patients whose main symptom is dysmenorrhea, the continuous use of COC, that is, without pausing, leads to amenorrhea, and this side effect should be considered. This course of treatment typically gives better results in the short term for the control of dysmenorrhea and improving the patient's quality of life [50].

2.1.2. Danazol

Danazol is an androgen that suppresses gonadotropins and acts by inhibiting ovulation. Its use in the treatment of endometriosis was first described in 1971 [51]. Several studies that compare this medication and GnRHa, combined oral contraceptives, or progestogens have shown the great effectiveness of this drug in the treatment of endometriosis. The drug promotes high patient satisfaction by improving the presenting symptoms, and consequently, has a positive impact on the quality of life [52,53]. However, the incidence of side effects with this drug is very high, and affect nearly 85% of users, as reported by Barbieri et al. in 1982 [52]. The principal adverse effects described are weight gain, edema, reduction in breast size, acne, hirsutism, oiliness of the skin, and changes in the voice [52], as well as having a potential negative influence on lipid metabolism by raising LDL-cholesterol and total cholesterol [54]. The adequate dosage is 600 mg/day. In a study comparing different doses of danazol (100, 200, 400, and 600 mg/day) Biberoglu and Behrman tried to determine the best dosage, and found that although a dose of 600 mg/day had the greatest incidence of side effects, it also had the best results in controlling dysmenorrhea, probably by induced amenorrhea [55].

2.1.3. GnRH Agonists (GnRHa)

Currently, GnRH agonists are considered to be the standard treatment for the pain associated with endometriosis. These agonists work by causing a state of hypoestrogenism. Their use in endometriosis was first described in a 1982 pilot study where 5 patients used this medication subcutaneously daily for 1 month and showed a significant clinical improvement [56]. Since then, several studies have been completed that compare this class of drugs with the other current treatments for endometriosis. GnRH agonists show an excellent therapeutical response with a significant improvement in the pelvic pain associated with endometriosis, a longer time before the recurrence of symptoms and the appearance of ovarian cystic lesions (endometriomas) [46,57-59]. The average time for the return of symptoms, such as dysmenorrhea, dispareunia, and cyclical pelvic pain varies greatly between 6 and 12 months after the end of treatment, but upon their return symptoms are less intense overall [60,61]. Therefore, we recommend the use of other forms of treatment after the completion of a course of GnRH agonist therapy, such as combined oral contraceptives, progestogens in any of the different routes of administration available, or non-hormonal anti-inflammatories.

However, the exact length of time this class of medication should be used in the clinical treatment of pain associated with endometriosis is not yet defined in the literature. Some authors recommend its use for six months, while others recommend its use for three months. The trend seems to be to use it for the shortest time necessary. Hornstein et al. compared the use of GnRHa treatment for three and six months in patients with pelvic pain associated with endometriosis, and demonstrated that there was no difference between the two periods of treatment with respect to improved pain relief, time until the reoccurrence of symptoms, or the need for later clinical or surgical treatment [62].

Another question that still generates uncertainty in the literature is the use of GnRHa after surgery for endometriosis as an adjuvant in the treatment of the disease. Several studies were conducted, but none generated conclusive data. In 1994, Parazzini et al. neither showed benefits of its use, nor observed an improvement in long term results [63]. Several years later, Hornstein et al. demonstrated that the improvement in pain and the delay in the recurrence of the disease were significantly greater after using these medications [59]. It seems that the clinic trend is towards the use of this medication, but for a period of time no longer than six months.

Clearly, the greatest inconvenience in using GnRHa to treat the pain associated with endometriosis is the occurrence of adverse secondary side effects due to hypoestrogenism. Among these side effects, hot flashes and vaginal drying are the primary effects, and are present in up to 90% of cases [64]. The less frequently cited side effects include chronic headaches, dizziness, emotional lability, acne, myalgia, edema, reduction in breast size, weight gain, reduction of libido, and insomnia [64]. Another large problem is the loss of bone mass that results due to the induced hypoestrogenism, which can vary between 3% to 6% after a six month period of use [65], and can be up to 12% after one year of use [66]. To prevent this bone loss and to minimize the side effects the Add-back therapy can be used, which consists of small doses of progestogens isolated or combined with estrogens during the GnRHa treatment [67]. Careful consideration should undertaken when considering a prescription for GnRH agonists to young women, who have yet to achieve peak bone mass.

2.2. Surgical Treatment of Endometriosis Associated with Pelvic Pain

The adequate evaluation of the effectiveness of different surgical techniques for the treatment of endometriosis associated with pelvic pain is difficult due to the small number of existing randomized and controlled studies.

Depending on the severity of the disease encountered, the practical ideal involves performing a diagnosis and surgical excision of the endometriosic foci during the same operation. Thus, obtaining pre-operative free and clarified consent, which covers the characterization of the procedure that potentially could be carried out, and the possible complications and rates of success, is recommended. There are no concrete data available that justify the prescription of hormonal treatment before the surgery with the aim of improving the success rate of the surgery [18].

Post-operative treatment with danazol or GnRH agonists for six months, reduces the pain associated with endometriosis and delays the recurrence of the disease, when compared to placebo or the standard therapy. However, post-operative treatment with combined oral contraceptives appears to not be effective [18].

The surgical treatment can be divided in two categories, conservative and radical treatments, with conservative treatments being those that preserve the fertility of the patient, and the radical treatments being those that involve a hysterectomy and a bilateral salpingo-oophorectomy, which is erroneously considered to be a definitive treatment for endometriosis. Such surgeries have recurrence rates of up to 10% for chronic pelvic pain [68]. Therefore, it seems inappropriate to consider this therapy as definitive. Hormone replacement therapy is recommended in cases where hysterectomy and bilateral salpingo-oophorectomy have been carried out in younger patients, but the best regimen for this is not well established. Thus, the prescription should be individualized and consider the risk-benefit ratio of hormone replacement therapy in each particular case.

2.2.1. Laparoscopy Versus Laparotomy

With current developments in the technology of laparoscopic devices, the effectiveness of this technique in the treatment of the patients with pelvic pain and endometriosis is unquestioned. Laparoscopic devices provide an excellent view of the pelvis, and consequently, of the endometrial lesions. Unfortunately, there is no concrete evidence available regarding which access route, laparoscopic or laparotomy, is the most effective in the treatment of disease and the related pain.

Several studies were conducted in attempts to compare the two surgical techniques for the treatment of women with pain and endometriosis. Their final goal was the evaluation of the time until the recurrence of dysmenorrhea, dyspareunia, and cyclic pain. In 1996, Crosignani et al. showed that patients with moderate or severe pelvic pain, and with stage IV endometriosis according to the American Society of Reproductive Medicine (ASRM) scale, the rates of recurrence of cyclic pain, dysmenorrheal, and dispareunia after 24 months of monitoring were statistically similar between the two techniques [69]. This data was corroborated by Busacca et al. [70] and Catalano et al. [71]. However, the laparoscopic approach has the advantages of less blood loss, less post-surgical recovery time, decreased post-operative pain, and decreased duration of hospitalization [72].

2.2.2. Laparoscopic Treatment

The destruction of lesions by coagulation, fulguration, or vaporization, or the excision of superficial lesions show similar results in improving the pelvic pain associated with endometriosis [73]. In 1997, Sutton et al. published a prospective and controlled study that demonstrated the destruction of the endometrial lesions has a beneficial effect when compared to laparoscopy alone, which does not destroy the lesions [74]. A similar result was disclosed by Abbott et al. [75] in 2004, which showed that superficial lesions should always be destroyed.

In regards to the approach for ovarian endometriomas in patients with pelvic pain, the main discussion is between the total removal of the pseudocapsule, or its drainage and coagulation. In 1998, Beretta et al. conducted a prospective and comparative study between these two laparoscopic techniques and showed that the recurrence of pelvic pain and the appearance of new endometriomas were greater in the group that underwent drainage and coagulation of the pseudocapsule, while both groups had similar rates of surgical complications [20]. These findings were corroborated by Saleh and Tulandi in 1999 [76], who showed a tendency in the literature toward the use of this technique, which also makes material available for anatomical-pathological analysis. However, Jones et al. published a comparative work in 2002 that showed the tendency of gynecologists in the United Kingdom to only perform the draining and coagulation of endometriomas, and showed equal recurrence rates of pelvic pain for both techniques [77].

In cases of deep infiltrative endometriosis, whether involving the rectum-vaginal septum, intestine, or bladder, the benefit of surgical treatment is very great. Chapron et al. showed that laparoscopy could be performed with success in the treatment of rectum-vaginal septum endometriosis, and provided a vast improvement in chronic pelvic pain with low rates of complication [78]. The laparoscopic approach was also used with great success by Abrão et al. for the resection of deep infiltrative endometriosis affecting the recto-sigmoid. These authors performed a segmentary resection of the recto-sigmoid, which had been infiltrated by endometriosis, via the vaginal route, while being assisted by laparoscopy [79]. We can conclude from these studies that the clinical improvement in the gynecological and intestinal symptoms that affect these women is significant with surgical treatment, and it should always be encouraged. However, this surgery should be performed by an experienced surgeon, and the patient should be aware of the possible complications [80].

Conclusion

The prevalence of endometriosis is extremely high, especially in patients with infertility and chronic pelvic pain. The bio-psycho-social impact of this intriguing and enigmatic disease is large both at the level of the individual and at the public health level. Treatment for the disease should always be individualized, and take into consideration not only the existing evidence on the effectiveness of different therapeutic regimes, but also the other influential variables in determining therapeutic success with the goal of promoting the greatest global improvement in the patient's quality of life. It is important to note that the controversies surrounding the treatment of endometriosis and its symptoms are innumerable, especially those related to the infertility that is associated with this disease. The following summary recommendations should be revised as additional controlled randomized clinical studies that involve appropriate patient populations generate more concrete and reliable evidence.

The suppression of ovarian function does not effectively improve fertility in patients with mild endometriosis, but the ablation of the lesions associated with adhesiolysis seems to be more effective than only performing diagnostic laparoscopy. The use of ovarian stimulation in conjunction with intrauterine insemination or IVF-ET can be considered, depending on other factors, such as the age of the patient, the duration of infertility, the presence of an associated masculine factor, and the response to other previously attempted therapies.

There is not enough evidence to determine if surgical excision improves gestation rates in cases of moderate or severe endometriosis.

In vitro fertilization (IVF) seems to be an adequate approach, especially in cases that involve several causes of infertility and/or the failure of other treatments. When the use of IVF is indicated, we recommend evaluating the possible use of GnRH agonists for 3 to 6 months prior to the use of controlled ovarian stimulation.

The suppression of ovarian function for 3 to 6 months in patients with confirmed cases of endometriosis has been verified to reduce the pain associated with the disease.

All of the medications studied, including medroxiprogesterone acetate, gestrinone, COC, danazol, and GnRH agonists are equally effective in pain relief, but their adverse side effects and their costs are different and must be taken into consideration when selecting a therapy.

The ablation of endometrial lesions reduces the pain associated with endometriosis, although it is less effective in milder cases of the disease.

Depending on the severity of the disease encountered, the ideal scenario involves performing the surgical diagnosis and excision of the endometriosic foci during the same operation. There are no concrete data that justify the prescription of hormonal treatment before surgery with regard to improving the success rate of the surgical approach.

Post-operative treatment with danazol or GnRH agonists for six months, reduces the pain associated with endometriosis and delays the recurrence of the disease when compared to the use of a placebo or the standard therapy. However, post-operative treatment with combined oral contraceptives appears not to be very effective.

The excision of endometriomas > 4 cm in diameter seems to improve the rate of natural fecundity after assisted reproduction procedures, as well as reduce the severity of the pain associated with endometriosis and delay the return of the disease.

References

[1] Borges, LS; Rosa e Silva, JC; Rosa e Silva, ACJS; Aguiar, FM; Poli Neto, OB; Candido dos Reis, FJ; Nogueira, AA. Evaluation of the diagnostic agreement between non invasive methods and endoscopy in infertility investigation. *Rev. Bras. Ginecol. Obstet.* 2005, 27, 401-5.

[2] Abrão, MS; Podgaec, S; Filho, BM; Ramos, LO; Pinotti, JA; de Oliveira, RM. The use of biochemical markers in the diagnosis of pelvic endometriosis. *Hum. Reprod.*, 1997, 12, 2523-7.

[3] Low, WY; Edelmann, RJ; Sutton, C. A psychological profile of patients in comparison to patients with pelvic pain of other origins. *J. Psychosom. Res.*, 1993, 37, 111-7.

[4] Chandra, A; Mosher, WD. The demograph of infertility and the use of medical care for infertility. *Infertil. Reprod. Med. Clin. North Am.,* 1994, 5, 283-96.

[5] Schwartz, D; Mayaux, MJ. Female fecundity as a function of age: results of artificial insemination in 2193 nulliparous women with azoozpermic husbands. Federation CECOS. *N. Engl. J. Med.*, 1982, 306, 404-6.

[6] Marcoux, S; Maheux, R; Berube, S. Laparoscopic surgery in infertile women with minimal or mild endometriosis. Canadian Collaborative Group on Endometriosis. *N. Engl. J. Med.*, 1997, 337, 217-22.

[7] Parazzini, F. Ablation of lesions or no treatment in minimal-mild endometriosis in infertile women: a randomized trial. Gruppo Italiano per lo Studio dell'Endometriosi. *Hum. Reprod.*, 1999, 14, 1332-4.

[8] Hughes, E; Fedorkow, D; Collins, J; Vandekerckhove, P. Ovulation suppression for endometriosis. *Cochrane Database Syst. Rev.*, 2003, (3), CD000155.

[9] Dicker, D; Goldman, GA; Ashkenazi, J; Feldberg, D; Voliovitz, I; Goldman, JA. The value of pre-treatment with long-term gonadotropin-releasing hormone (GnRH) analogue in IVF-ET therapy of severe endometriosis., 1990, 5, 418-20.

[10] Marcus, SF; Edwards, RG. High rates of pregnancy after long term down regulation of women with severe endometriosis. *Am. J. Obstet. Gynecol.*, 1994, 171, 812-7.

[11] Surrey, ES; Silverberg, KM; Surrey, MW; Schoolcraft, WB. The effect of prolonged GnRH agonist therapy on an in vitro fertilization-embryo transfer cycle outcome in patients with endometriosis. *Fertil. Steril.*, 2002, 78, 699-704.

[12] Sallan, HN; Garcia-Velasco, JA; Dias, S; Arici, A. Long-term pituitary down-regulation before in vitro fertilization (IVF) for women with endometriosis. *Cochrane Database Syst. Rev.*, 2006, 25(1), CD004635.

[13] Allaire, C. Endometriosis and infertility. *J. Reprod. Med.*, 2006, 51, 164-8.

[14] Jacobson, TZ; Barlow, DH; Koninckx, PR; Olive, D; Farquhar, C. Laparoscopic surgery for subfertility associated with endometriosis. *Cochrane Database Syst. Rev.*, 2002, 22, CD001398.

[15] Adamson, GD; Hurd, SJ; Pasta, DJ; Rodriguez, BD. Laparoscopic endometriosis treatment: is it better? *Fertil. Steril.*, 1993, 59, 35-44.

[16] Guzick, DS; Silliman, NP; Adamson, GD; Buttram, VC; Jr; Canis, M; Malinak, LR. Prediction of pregnancy in infertile women based on the American Society for Reproductive Medicine's revised classification of endometriosis. *Fertil. Steril.*, 1997, 67, 822-9.

[17] Osuga, Y; Koga, K; Tsutsumi, O; Yano, T; Maruyama, M; Kugu, K. Role of laparoscopy in the treatment of endometriosis-associated infertility. *Gynecol. Obstet. Invest.*, 2002, 53, 33-9.

[18] Kennedy, S; Bergqvist, A; Chapron, C; D'Hooghe, T; Dunselman, G; Greb, R. ESHRE guideline for the diagnosis and treatment of endometriosis. *Hum. Reprod.*, 2005, 20, 2698–704.

[19] Hart, R; Hickey, M; Maouris, P; Buckett, W; Garry, R. Excisional surgery versus ablative surgery for ovarian endometriomata: a Cochrane Review. *Hum. Reprod.*, 2005, 20, 3000-7.

[20] Beretta, P; Franchi, M; Ghezzi, F; Busacca, M; Zupi, E; Bolis, P. Randomized clinical trial of two laparoscopic treatments of endometriomas: cystectomy versus drainage and coagulation. *Fertil. Steril.*, 1998, 70, 1176-80.

[21] Chapron, C; Vercellini, P; Barakat, H; Vieira, M; Dubuisson, JB. Management of ovarian endometriomas. *Hum. Reprod. Update.*, 2002, 8, 6-7.

[22] Vercellini, P; Chapron, C; De Giorgi, O; Consonni, D; Frontino, G; Crosignani, PG. Coagulation or excision of ovarian endometriomas? *Am. J. Obstet. Gynecol.*, 2003, 188, 606-10.

[23] Nargund, G; Cheng, WC; Parsons, J. The impact of ovarian cystectomy on ovarian response to stimulation during in-vitro fertilization cycles. *Hum. Reprod.*, 1996, 11, 81-3.

[24] Loh, FH; Tan, AT; Kumar, J; Ng, SC. Ovarian response after laparoscopic ovarian cystectomy for endometriotic cysts in 132 monitored cycles. *Fertil. Steril.*, 1999, 72, 316-21.

[25] Hachisuga, T; Kawarabayashi, T. Histopathological analysis of laparoscopically treated ovarian endometriotic cysts with special reference to loss of follicles. *Hum. Reprod.*, 2002, 17, 432-5.

[26] Geber, S; Ferreira, DP; Spyer Prates, LF; Sales, L; Sampaio, M. Effects of previous ovarian surgery for endometriosis on the outcome of assisted reproduction treatment. *Reprod. Biomed. Online*, 2002, 5, 162-6.

[27] Ho, HY; Lee, RK; Hwu, YM; Lin, MH; Su, JT; Tsai, YC. Poor response of ovaries with endometrioma previously treated with cystectomy to controlled ovarian hyperstimulation. *J. Assist. Reprod. Genet.*, 2002, 19, 507-11.

[28] Somigliana, E; Ragni, G; Benedetti, F; Borroni, R; Vegetti, W; Crosignani, PG. Does laparoscopic excision of endometriotic ovarian cysts significantly affect ovarian reserve? Insights from IVF cycles. *Hum. Reprod.*, 2003, 18, 2450-3.

[29] Bianchi, S; Busacca, M; Agnoli, B; Candiani, M; Calia, C; Vignali, M. Effects of 3 month therapy with danazol after laparoscopic surgery for stage III/IV endometriosis: a randomized study. *Hum. Reprod.*, 1999, 14, 1335-7.

[30] Busacca, M; Somigliana, E; Bianchi, S; De Marinis, S; Calia, C; Candiani, M. Post-operative GnRH analogue treatment after conservative surgery for symptomatic endometriosis stage III-IV: a randomized controlled trial. *Hum. Reprod.*, 2001, 16, 2399-402.

[31] Vercellini, P; Crosignani, PG; Fadini, R; Radici, E; Belloni, C; Sismondi, P. A gonadotrophin-releasing hormone agonist compared with expectant management after conservative surgery for symptomatic endometriosis. *Br. J. Obstet. Gynaecol.*, 1999, 106, 672-7.

[32] Chaffkin, LM; Nulsen, JC; Luciano, AA; Metzger, DA. A comparative analysis of the cycle fecundity rates associated with combined human menopausal gonadotrophin (hMG) and intrauterine insemination (IUI) versus either hMG or IUI alone. *Fertil. Steril.*, 1991, 55, 252-7.

[33] Deaton, JL; Gibson, M; Blackmer, KM; Nakajima, ST; Badger, GJ; Brumsted, JR. A randomized, controlled trial of clomiphene citrate and intrauterine insemination in couples with unexplained infertility or surgically corrected endometriosis. *Fertil. Steril.*, 1990, 54, 1083-8.

[34] Barnhart, K; Dunsmoor-Su, R; Coutfaris, C. Effect of endometriosis on in vitro fertilization. *Fertil. Steril.*, 2002, 77, 1148-55.

[35] Kistner, R. The use of newer progestins in the treatment of endometriosis. *Am. J. Obstet. Gynecol.*, 1958, 75, 264-78.

[36] Luciano, A; Turskoy, R; Carleo, J. Evaluation of oral medroxyprogesterone acetate in the treatment of endometriosis. *Obstet. Gynecol.*, 1988, 72, 323-7.

[37] Harrison, R; Barry-Kinsella, C. Efficacy of medroxyprogesterone treatment in infertile women with endometriosis, A prospective, randomized, placebocontrolled study. *Fertil. Steril.*, 2000, 74, 24-30.

[38] Vercellini, P; De Giorgi, O; Oldani, S; Cortesi, I; Panazza, S; Crosignani, P. Depot medroxyprogesterone acetate versus an oral contraceptive combined with very low-

dose danazol for long-term treatment of pelvic pain associated with endometriosis. *Am. J. Obstet. Gynecol.*, 1996, 175, 396-401.

[39] Nieto, A; Tacuri, C; Serra, M; Keller, J; Cortés-Prieto, J. Long-term follow-up of endometriosis after two different therapies (gestrinone and buserelin). *Clin. Exp. Obstet. Gynecol.*, 1996, 23, 198-204.

[40] Gestrinone versus a gonadotropin-releasing hormone agonist for the treatment of pelvic pain associated with endometriosis: A multicenter, randomized, doubleblind study. Gestrinone Italian Study Group. *Fertil. Steril.,* 1996, 66, 911-9.

[41] Fedele, L; Arcaini, L; Bianchi, S; Baglioni, A; Vercellini, P. Comparison of cyproterone acetate and danazol in the treatment of pelvic pain associated with endometriosis. *Obstet. Gynecol.*, 1989, 73, 1000-4.

[42] Muneyyirci-Delale, O; Karacan, M. Effect of norethindrone acetate in the treatment of symptomatic endometriosis. *Int. J. Fertil. Womens Med.*, 1998; 43, 24-7.

[43] Yisa, SB; Okenwa, AA; Husemeyer, RP. Treatment of pelvic endometriosis with etonogestrel subdermal implant (Implanon). *J. Fam. Plann. Reprod. Health Care.,* 2005, 31, 67-70.

[44] Vercellini, P; Aimi, G; Panazza, S; De Giorgi, O; Pesole, A; Crosignani, PG. A levonorgestrel-releasing intrauterine system for the treatment of dysmenorrhea associated with endometriosis: a pilot study. *Fertil. Steril.*, 1999,72, 505-8.

[45] Fedele, L; Bianchi, S; Zanconato, G; Portuese, A; Raffaelli, R. Use of levonorgestrel-releasing intrauterine device in the treatment of rectovaginal endometriosis. *Fertil. Steril.*, 2001, 75, 485-8.

[46] Petta, CA; Ferriani, RA; Abrao, MS; Hassan, D; Rosa e Silva, JC; Podgaec, S; Bahamondes, L. Randomized clinical trial of a levonorgestrel-releasing intrauterine system and a depot GnRH analogue for the treatment of chronic pelvic pain in women with endometriosis. *Hum. Reprod.*, 2005, 20, 1993-8.

[47] Rosa e Silva, AC; Rosa e Silva, JC; Nogueira, AA; Petta, CA; Abrao, MS; Ferriani, RA. The levonorgestrel-releasing intrauterine device reduces CA-125 serum levels in patients with endometriosis. *Fertil. Steril.,* 2006, 86, 742-4.

[48] Vercellini, P; Trespidi, L; Colombo, A; Vendola, N; Marchini, M; Crosignani, P. A gonadotropin-releasing hormone agonist versus a low-dose oral contraceptive for pelvic pain associated with endometriosis. *Fertil. Steril.*, 1993, 60, 75-9.

[49] Muzii, L; Marana, R; Caruana, P; Catalano, G; Margutti, F; Panici, P. Postoperative administration of monophasic combined oral contraceptives after laparoscopic treatment of ovarian endometriomas: A prospective, randomized trial. *Am. J. Obstet. Gynecol.*, 2000, 183, 588-92.

[50] Edelman, A; Gallo, M; Jensen, J; Nichols, M; Schulz, K; Grimes, D. Continuous or extended cycle vs. cyclic use of combined oral contraceptives for contraception. *Cochrane Database Syst. Rev.*, 2005, 20(3), CD004695.

[51] Greenblatt, R; Dmowski, W; Mahesh, VB; Scholer, H. Clinical studies with an antigonadotropin-danazol. *Fertil. Steril.*, 1971, 22, 102-12.

[52] Barbieri, R; Evans, S; Kistner, R. Danazol in the the treatment of endometriosis: Analysis of 100 cases with a 4-year follow-up. *Fertil. Steril.*, 1982, 37, 737-46.

[53] Henzl, M; Corson, S; Moghissi, K; Buttram, V; Berqvist, C; Jacobson, J. Administration of nasal nafarelin as compared with oral danazol for endometriosis. A multicenter double-blind comparative clinical trial. *N. Engl. J. Méd.,* 1988, 318, 485-9.

[54] Cirkel, U; Ochs, H; Schneider, H. A randomized, comparative trial of triptorelin (D-Trp6-LHRH) and danazol in the treatment of endometriosis. *Eur. J. Obstet. Gynecol. Reprod. Biol.,* 1995, 59, 61-9.

[55] Biberoglu, K; Behrman, S. Dosage aspects of danazol therapy in endometriosis: Short-term and long-term effectiveness. *Am. J. Obstet. Gynecol.*, 1981, 139, 645-54.

[56] Meldrum, D; Chang, R; Lu, J; Vale, W; Rivier, J; Judd, H. "Medical oophorectomy" using a long-acting GnRH agonist-A possible new approach to the treatment of endometriosis. *J. Clin. Endocrinol. Metab.*, 1982;54, 1081-3.

[57] Dlugi, A; Miller, J; Knittle, J. Lupron Study Group. Lupron depot (leuprolide acetate for depot suspension) in the treatment of endometriosis: A randomized, placebo-controlled, double-blind study. *Fertil. Steril.*, 1990, 54, 419-27.

[58] Ling, F. for the Pelvic Pain Study Group. Randomized controlled trial of depot leuprolide in patients with chronic pelvic pain and clinically suspected endometriosis. Pelvic Pain Study Group. *Obstet. Gynecol.*, 1999, 93, 51-8.

[59] Hornstein, M; Hemmings, R; Yuzpe, A; Heinrichs, W. Use of nafarelin versus placebo after reductive laparoscopic surgery for endometriosis. *Fertil. Steril.*, 1997, 68, 860-4.

[60] Jacobson, J; Harris, S; Bullingham, R. Low-dose intranasal nafarelin for the treatment of endometriosis. *Acta Obstet. Gynecol. Scand.*, 1994, 73, 144-50.

[61] Fedele, L; Bianchi, S; Bocciolone, L; Di Nola, G; Franchi, D. Buserelin acetate in the treatment of pelvic pain associated with minimal and mild endometriosis: a controlled study. *Fertil. Steril.*, 1993, 59, 516-21.

[62] Hornstein, M; Yuzpe, A; Burry, K; Heinrichs, L; Buttram V, Jr; Orwoll, E. Prospective randomized double-blind trial of 3 versus 6 months of nafarelin therapy for endometriosis associated pelvic pain. *Fertil. Steril.*, 1995, 63, 955-62.

[63] Parazzini, F; Fedele, L; Busacca, M. Postsurgical medical treatment of advanced endometriosis: results of a randomized clinical trial. *Am. J. Obstet. Gynecol.,* 1994, 171, 1205-7.

[64] Henzl, M; Kwei, L. Efficacy and safety of nafarelin in the treatment of endometriosis. *Am. J. Obstet. Gynecol.,* 1990, 162, 570-4.

[65] Scialli, A; Jestila, K; Simon, J. Leuprolide acetate and bone mineral density measured by quantitative digitized radiography. *Fertil. Steril.*, 1993, 59, 674-6.

[66] Mukherjee, T; Barad, D; Turk, R; Freeman, R. A randomized, placebo-controlled study on the effect of cyclic intermittent etidronate therapy on the bone mineral density changes associated with six months of gonadotropin-releasing hormone agonist treatment. *Am. J. Obstet. Gynecol.*, 1996, 175, 105-9.

[67] Surrey, E; the Add-Back Consensus Working Group. Add-back therapy and gonadotropin-releasing hormone agonists in the treatment of patients with endometriosis: can a consensus be reached? Add-Back Consensus Working Group., *Fertil. Steril.* 1999, 71, 420-4.

[68] Clayton, RD; Hawe, JA; Love, JC; Wilkinson, N; Garry, R. Recurrent pain after hysterectomy and bilateral salpingo-oophorectomy for endometriosis: Evaluation of laparoscopic excision of residual endometriosis. *Br. J. Obstet. Gynaecol.*, 1999, 106, 740-4.

[69] Crosignani, PG; Vercellini, P; Biffignandi, F; Costantini, W; Cortesi, I; Imparato, E. Laparoscopy versus laparotomy in conservative surgical treatment for severe. *Fertil. Steril.*, 1996, 66, 706-11.

[70] Busacca, M; Fedele, L; Bianchi, S. Surgical treatment of recurrent endometriosis: laparotomy versus laparoscopy. *Hum. Reprod.*, 1998, 13, 2271-4.

[71] Catalano, GF; Marana, R; Caruana, P; Muzii, L; Mancuso, S. Laparoscopy versus microsurgery by laparotomy for excision of ovarian cysts in patients with moderate or severe endometriosis. *J. Am. Assoc. Gynecol. Laparosc.*, 1996, 3, 267-70.

[72] Ekstein, P; Szold, A; Sagie, B; Werbin, N; Klausner, JM; Weinbroum, AA. Laparoscopic surgery may be associated with severe pain and high analgesia requirements in the immediate postoperative period. *Ann. Surg.*, 2006, 243, 41-6.

[73] Wright, J; Lotfallah, H; Jones, K; Lovell, D. A randomized trial of excision versus ablation for mild endometriosis. *Fertil. Steril.*, 2005, 83, 1830-6.

[74] Sutton, CJ; Pooley, AS; Ewen, SP; Haines, P. Follow-up report on a randomized controlled trial of laser laparoscopy in the treatment of pelvic pain associated with minimal to moderate endometriosis. *Fertil. Steril.*, 1997, 68, 1070-4.

[75] Abbott, J; Hawe, J; Hunter, D; Holmes, M; Finn, P; Garry, R. Laparoscopic excision of endometriosis: a randomized, placebo-controlled trial. *Fertil. Steril.*, 82, 878- 84.

[76] Saleh, A; Tulandi, T. Reoperation after laparoscopic treatment for ovarian endometriomas by excision and by fenestration. *Fertil. Steril.*, 1999, 72, 322-4.

[77] Jones, KD; Fan, A; Sutton, CJG. The ovarian endometrioma: why is it so poorly managed? *Hum. Reprod.*, 2002, 17, 845-9.

[78] Chapron, C; Jacob, S; Dubuisson, JB; Vieira, M; Liaras, E; Fauconnier, A. Laparoscopically assisted vaginal management of deep endometriosis infiltrating the rectovaginal septum. *Acta Obstet. Gynecol. Scand.*, 2001, 80, 349-54.

[79] Abrao, MS; Sagae, UE; Gonzales, M; Podgaec, S; Dias, JA; Jr. Treatment of rectosigmoid endometriosis by laparoscopically assisted vaginal rectosigmoidectomy. *Int. J. Gynaecol. Obstet.*, 2005, 91, 27-31.

[80] Dubernard, G; Piketty, M; Rouzier, R; Houry, S; Bazot, M; Darai, E. Quality of life after laparoscopic colorectal resection for endometriosis. *Hum. Reprod.*, 2006, 21, 1243-7.

Index

D

E

F

G

H

I

K

L

M

N

O

P

Q

R

S